SpringerBriefs in Statistics

For further volumes:
http://www.springer.com/series/8921

Carlos N. Bouza-Herrera

Handling Missing Data
in Ranked Set Sampling

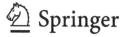 Springer

Carlos N. Bouza-Herrera
Facultad de Matemática y Computación
Universidad de La Habana
Havana
Cuba

ISSN 2191-544X   ISSN 2191-5458   (electronic)
ISBN 978-3-642-39898-8   ISBN 978-3-642-39899-5   (eBook)
DOI 10.1007/978-3-642-39899-5
Springer Heidelberg New York Dordrecht London

Library of Congress Control Number: 2013944885

Mathematics Subject Classification (2010): 62D05, 62F05, 62F10, 62Pxx, 62F40

Printed on acid-free paper

Springer is part of Springer Science+Business Media (www.springer.com)

To my jewels:
Gemayqzel, for being the brilliant apple of
my eyes
Sira María, the constant and shining support
of my heart
Bernarda Dulce, the precious diamond of our
lifes

Preface

Usage is the best language teacher.

Quintilianus

The use of random sampling sustains the development of current statistical theory. In many cases it is necessary to have some control of the units to be selected. The solution in classic sampling is to use stratification, clustering, unequal probabilities of selection, etc. Ranked Set Sampling (RSS) is a new method of selection of samples. RSS allows controlling the selection procedure, as the sample will contain units in which the values of the variables of interest are spread throughout the interval of possible values. The sample consists of units with different ranks. Ranks are assigned using some auxiliary information; the judgment of experts is a particular case.

RSS is a kind of stratification. Hence, using this design instead of simple random sampling with replacement means that a gain in accuracy is straightforwardly achieved. It is sustained by the fact that each strata consists of population units with the same rank. The statistical properties of order statistics allow deriving the properties of RSS-based estimators. One of the main consequences of the study of RSS methods is determining formulas for evaluating the gains in accuracy as well as relative precision measures.

From the proposal of McIntyre (1952) to the book of Chen et al. (2004), the study of particular RSS strategies has produced a large number of papers and a body of models has formed an alternative theory of sampling. The number of theoretical papers and applications of RSS is growing. One of the usual problems in sampling applications is the presence of non-sampling errors. The effects of ranking errors have been studied. This work deals with the problems derived by no responses. RSS models after subsampling the non-respondents and imputation procedures are studied.

The aim of this book is quite modest; it attempts to be a systematic exposition of all that is contained in the literature on RSS in the area of missing observations. In writing this book, I tried to produce a text that is as simple as possible. My aim is to spread awareness of the potentialities of RSS. I am hopeful that this oeuvre will trigger additional theoretical research, as well as provide tools for practical applications, when non-sampling errors are present and an RSS model is used. Hence my torch was Quintilianus maxima: consuetudo certissima est loquendi magistra.

I am deeply indebted to my family for their invaluable and kind support. I give my hearty thanks to the staff of SpringerBriefs, Evelyn Best, Eva Hiripi, and Veronika Rosteck, for their responsiveness through the entire Editorial Process, and, last but not least, to the specialists whose comments and suggestions allowed improving the initial version of this book.

La Habana, Cuba, October 29, 2012   Carlos N. Bouza-Herrera

References

McIntyre, G. A. (1952). A method of unbiased selective sampling using ranked sets. *Australian Journal of Agricultural Research, 3*, 385–390.
Chen, Z., Bai, Z., & Sinha, B. K. (2004). *Ranked set sampling: Theory and applications.* Lectures Notes in Statistics, (p.176). New York: Springer.

Contents

Chapter 1
Missing Observations and Data Quality Improvement

Abstract Missing data is a well-recognized problem which arises in statistical inferences and data analysis. We address different possible ways to handle missing data, to ameliorate its effect on the reliability and accuracy of survey-based inferences. Subsampling the non-respondents and imputation of missing values, are considered as methods for dealing with non-responses. This book presents the work developed on Ranked Set Sampling (RSS) in dealing with missing data. RSS is a relatively new sampling design. This chapter may be considered as an introduction to the rest of the oeuvre.

Keywords Non respondent · Imputation · Randomized responses · Simple random sampling · Ranked set sampling

> *What the caterpillar calls the end of the world, the rest of the world calls a butterfly.*
>
> Lao Tse

1.1 Missing Observations and Data Quality

Consider a finite population U of size N from which a simple random sample s, of size n, is drawn with replacement. Full response surveys are rare situations. In sample surveys it is common that some units are missing at the first measurement attempt. Let the characteristic under study determine a variable Y. For each $i \in U$ we can determine the value of Y_i. When some units do not provide information we have that the sample is divided into two subsets.

$$s_r = \{i \in U \mid \text{the response } Y_i \text{ is obtained}\}, \; s_{rn}$$
$$= \{i \in U \mid \text{the response } Y_i \text{ is not obtained}\}$$

An estimate obtained from s_r only is biased and may be misleading.

C. N. Bouza-Herrera, *Handling Missing Data in Ranked Set Sampling*, SpringerBriefs in Statistics, DOI: 10.1007/978-3-642-39899-5_1, © The Author(s) 2013

Sampling survey practice compromises fixing a series of considerations. Before a survey can be developed many factors must be taken into account. Concepts, definitions, methods of collecting and processing data must be determined beforehand. They determine a working system, which is shaped by the aims of the survey and some key decisions, determined by the statisticians, are involved in the design of the inquiry.

It is common that data are not collected for all the units in the sample. Data can be missing for a part of the population and different problems arise when conclusions are to be taken using statistical methods. For different reasons the units may be unavailable, when they are going to be measured, or refuse giving information. Missing data is the common name for all cases in which the value of the variable of interest is not obtained.

The existence of missing values is one of the most pervasive problems in data analysis because they are present in many research activities. The seriousness of the problem depends on the pattern of the missing data, the distribution of missingness, how much is missing, and why it is missing. Missing data are widespread in social science surveying, as the interviewees are unable or unwilling to answer some questions. But it is a recurrent issue not only in sampling human populations. It is also a common problem in psychological, medical research and, recently, informatics is also dealing with it. The decision about how to handle missing data is very important as it affects the reliability and accuracy of the inferences about the population of interest. Missing data rates are a measure of the level of unit response. Frequently, surveyors use them as an indirect indicator of the quality of the data.

Missing data in survey research are present because:

1. An element in the target population U is not included on the survey's sampling frame (non-coverage);
2. A sampled element does not participate in the survey (total nonresponse);
3. A unit in the sample fails to provide acceptable responses (item or unit nonresponse).

Weighting adjustments are often used to compensate for non-coverage and total nonresponse (NR). Subsampling among the nonrespondents or imputation methods are used for dealing with unit nonresponse. A variety of methods have been developed trying to compensate for missing data. The magnitude of nonresponse (NR) bias may be partially assessed, Särndal and Lundstrom (2005) for a detailed discussion on this issue. Data quality often needs to subsample nonrespondents for following-up.

The existence of nonresponse in surveys induces a non-observational error reflecting an unsuccessful attempt to obtain the desired (needed) information from a selected unit. Unit nonresponse is a failure to obtain any data from a sample unit. Item nonresponse is defined when we deal with the measurement of k variables and some of them are not measured. Usually the values of Y in the nonrespondents are in general not similar to the values of it in the respondents. Hence, ignoring them is not a good decision. Many studies have attempted to determine if there is a difference between respondents and nonrespondents. Some researchers have reported that people who respond to surveys answer questions differently than those who do not. Others have found that late responders answer differently than early responders, and that the differences may be due to the different levels of interest in the subject matter or to avoid being identified as belonging to a stigmatized group.

Generally surveyors decide to subsample the nonrespondents when the response rate is lower than expected and to interview them all is too costly. Another reason is that nonresponse constitutes an important potential source of bias. Subsampling the nonrespondents allows also studying the reasons for avoiding responding. Commonly a representative subsample of nonrespondents is taken (those units generating missing data) and it is used for inferring about them. The work of Hansen and Hurwitz (1946), pioneering the treatment of nonresponse, suggested a double sampling scheme for estimating population mean. Different authors have discussed approaches for subsampling the nonrespondents; see Srinath (1971) and Bouza (1981).

There is an extensive literature concerning missing data, much of which has focused on missing outcomes. The best way to deal with nonresponses (NR) is to prevent its happening. It determines that the surveyor must spend the needed time in designing surveys and building previsions, for dealing with nonresponse. To design experiments to reduce nonresponse is advisable. When NR are present it is advisable to use existent information to predict the missing data. Then a model is to be used to predict values for the nonresponse and imputation can be used for adjusting for item nonresponse.

Imputation means to substitute missing data with plausible values. Some practitioners consider that it solves the missing-data problem. But it must use some model. A naïve method, subjective evaluations or unsound modeling imputation methods may generate serious additional problems. The processes of imputation and analysis should be guided by common sense. If not, we will be dealing with bad estimates, false standard errors, and unreliable hypothesis tests. See Little and Rubin (2002) for a documented discussion. In some cases, good estimates can be obtained by substituting the missing observation by some supposedly close value of Y or by using some weighting estimation procedures. The usual approach in survey sampling is based in imposing a probability model on the complete data (observed and missing values). Surveyors are aware that real data are seldom described by convenient models. The theory of imputation for missing data requires that imputations be made conditional on the sampling design. It is advisable that an imputation model should produce imputation values, which are at least approximately compatible with the analyses to be performed on the imputed datasets. For example it must preserve the associations or relationships among items. For modeling we should consider that exists the Bernoulli variable.

$$R_i = \begin{cases} 1 \text{ if unit i responds} \\ 0 \text{ otherwise} \end{cases}, \ i = 1, \ldots, N$$

Then, at least, an additional source of randomness is present in imputation procedures. Another approach is to consider the set of simulation methods that have appeared in the statistical literature for imputing. These methods, known as Markov Chain Monte Carlo (MCMC), are being increasingly considered but rely on a knowledge of the phenomena under study, which is uncommon in survey sampling applications.

1.2 Ranked Set Sample in the Presence of Missing Data

Chapter 2 is intended to provide the reader with an introduction to Ranked Set Sampling (RSS). It was introduced by McIntyre (1952) to estimate the pasture yields. Recently attention is being paid to the basic theory of RSS. The literature in the subject presents new techniques and approaches. RSS is a method of collecting data that improves estimation by utilizing the sampler's judgment or auxiliary information about the relative sizes of the sampling units. The procedure involves randomly drawing independently m sets of m units each from the population. Hence, the selection of the units evaluated takes into account the order of them in the combined m samples. The units in each set are cheaply ranked. From the first set of m units, the unit ranked lowest is measured; from the second set of m units, the unit ranked second lowest is measured and the process is continued until from the m- th set of m units the m -th ranked unit is measured. A sample of size n is obtained by repeating the procedure r (r $\geq$ 1) times independently for obtaining n = mr. RSS is an alternative to simple random sampling which has been shown to outperform simple random sampling (SRS) in many situations. RSS outperforms SRSWR in terms of efficiency, as it has a smaller variance in estimating, and increases the power in testing hypothesis, especially for nonparametric ones. As a result it provides the same accuracy using smaller sample sizes than the SRS alternatives. Auxiliary variables are commonly used in survey sampling. They may be derived from various sources as registers, administrative sources subjective evaluation of the interest variable etc. In RSS the sampled units are ranked using some non-costly auxiliary variable. The auxiliary variable X must be related with Y. We may also rank using judgments. We will deal with the estimation of the population mean.

The literature addressing how to deal with missing data can be divided by the need of obtaining information from the nonresponses and to diminish the amount of missing data.

In Chap. 3 we will consider subsampling among the nonrespondents for dealing with missing data. The usual theory is presented in text books for simple random sampling, see (Cochran 1997), Hedayat and Sinha (1992). The use of ranked set sample is considered and models are discussed. Two problems are posed and studied at large:

1. Dealing with nonresponses in RSS.
2. Using RSS for subsampling among the nonrespondents using the information at hand in the population or provided in the first attempt for measuring Y.

The existence of nonresponse motivates to select a subsample among the nonrespondents or imputing the values of the interest variables on the nonrespondents. The use of imputation techniques for dealing with missing information is a theme of actuality. See for example Bouza and Al-Omari (Bouza and Al-Omari 2011a, b), Chang and Huang (2001), Fitzenberger et al. (2005), Rueda and González (2004), Young-Jae (2005), Singh and Deo (2003), Singh and Horn (2000), Toutenburg et al. (2008) and Zou and Feng (1998).

Chapter 4 is concerned with the use of imputation in RSS. The missing values can be identified with no-responses on a certain order statistic. Hence we have some missing observations but in general there are replicas of them if the RSS procedure is repeated r times (cycles) to have n = rm observations, for example. Different imputation procedures used in survey sampling are visited and developed for RSS. To study the properties of imputation-based estimators, are often considered through the consideration of a superpopulation model, the sampling mechanism generating the sample, the variable response mechanism and the imputation mechanism. In survey sampling practice it is advisable to use simple relations between the variable of interest Y and the auxiliary one X. In RSS as we may use X for ranking which seems to increase the accuracy. Some ratio relations are the simpler models. A study of the existent models is developed at large. Other models are also developed and discussed.

Chapter 5 is devoted to analyzing different numerical experiments planned for evaluating the efficiency of RSS-based estimators. They permit comparing SRSWR and the RSS alternatives. Some experiments are simulations using certain friendly probability distribution functions. The rest use real-life data and artificial populations are constituted. Monte Carlo experiments evaluate the behavior of the efficiency of the estimators.

References

Bouza, C. N. & Al-Omari, A. (2011a). Ratio imputation of missing data in ranked set sampling.accepted by Statistics, GSTA-2011-0026.r2. Nasr: Hindawi Publishing Corporation.

Bouza, C. N., & Al-Omari, A. (2011b). Imputation methods of missing data for estimating the population mean using simple random sampling with known correlation coefficient. *Quality and Quantity,*. doi:10.1007/S11135-011-9522-1.

Bouza, C. N. (1981). On the problem of subsample fraction in case of non response. (Spanish). *Trabolhos Estadisca Investigation Operation., 32,* 30–36.

Chang, H. J., & Huang, K. (2001). Ratio estimation in survey sampling when some observations are missing. *International Journal of Information and Management Sciences, 12,* 1.

Cochran, W.G. (1997). Sampling techniques. N. york: Wiley.

Fitzenberger, B., Osikominu, A., & Väolter, R. (2005). Imputation rules to improve the education variable in the IAB employment subsample. *ZEW Discussion Paper* 05–10, Mannheim.

Hansen, M. H., & Hurwitz, W. N. (1946). The problem of non-response in sample surveys. *Journal of the American Statistical Association, 41,* 517–529.

Hedayat, A. S., & Sinha, B. K. (1992). *Design and inference in finite population sampling.* New York: Wiley.

McIntyre, G. A. (1952). A method of unbiased selective sampling using ranked sets. *Australian Journal of Agricultural Research, 3,* 385–390.

Särndal, C. E., & Lundstrom, S. (2005). *Estimation in surveys with non-response.* New York: Wiley.

Singh, S. & Horn, S. (2000): Compromised imputation in survey sampling. METRIKA, *51,* 267–276.

Singh, S., & Deo, B. (2003). Imputation by power transformation. *Statistical Papers, 44,* 555–579.

Srinath, K. P. (1971). Multi-phase sampling in non-response problems. *Jounal of the American Statistical Association, 66,* 583–589.

Toutenburg, V., Srivastava, K., & Shalab, H. (2008). Amputation versus imputation of missing values through ratio method in sample surveys. *Statistical Papers, 49,* 237–247.

Young-Jae, M. (2005). Monotonicity conditions and inequality imputation for sample and non-response problems. *Economic Review, 24,* 175–194.

Zou, G. & Feng, S. (1998). Sample rotation method with missing data.Paper presented at the 4th ICSA Statistical Conference, Kunming, China.

Chapter 2
Sampling Using Ranked Sets: Basic Concepts

Abstract Simple random sampling is the kernel of sampling theory. The basic theory of statistical inference is supported by the assumption of using samples selected by means of this design. During the last decade Ranked Set Sampling has appeared as a challenge to this design. It is implemented by selecting units with replacement and the sampled units are ordered (ranked). Each order statistic is observed once. This process can be repeated if needed to observe various realizations of each order statistic. A review of the most significant results is developed in this chapter, taking into account the modeling of missing data.

Keywords Estimation · Ranking · Order statistics · Unbiasedness · Accuracy · Precision

> *God grant me the serenity to accept the things I cannot change; courage to change the things I can; and wisdom to know the difference.*
> From the Serenity Prayer (Copyright © The AA Grapevine, Inc. (January, 1950). Reprinted with permission. Permission to reprint The AA Grapevine, Inc., copyrighted material in this publication does not in any way imply affiliation with or endorsement by either Alcoholics Anonymous or The AA Grapevine, Inc.).

2.1 Introduction

Ranked set sampling (RSS) was first proposed by McIntyre (1952). He used this model for estimating the mean of pasture yields. This design appeared as a useful technique for improving the accuracy of the estimation of means. This fact was affirmed by McIntyre but a mathematical proof of it was settled by Takahashi-Wakimoto (1968). An interesting paper is Yanagawa (2000) where and account of

Wakinoto's contributions is made. In many situations the statistician deals with the need of combining some control and/or implementing some flexibility in the use of a random-based sample. This is a common problem in the study of environmental and medical studies, for example. In these cases the researcher generally has abundant and accurate information on the population units. It is related with the variable of interest Y and to rank the units using this information is cheap. The RSS procedure is based on the selection of m independent samples, not necessarily of the same size, by using simple random sampling (SRS) with replacement (SRSWR). The sampled units are ranked and the selection of the units evaluated takes into account the order of them in the combined m samples. The proposal of McIntyre (1952) was to use a prediction of Y. After some experiences with its application the lack of a coherent statistical theory appeared as an interesting theme of study by theoretical statisticians. An important role was played by Hall-Dell (1966) who established that RSS was more efficient than SRSWR for estimating the population mean derived from a large study of sampling forage yields. The interest for RSS in applications is reflected not only in initial papers but in the orientation of a series of papers to practice. See for example Chen (1999), Demir-Singh (2000), Kaur et.al. (1997), Hall-Dell (1966) for examples. The interest in the development of a new statistical theory using RSS can be illustrated by the contributions of Adatia (2000), Abu-Dayyeh and Muttlak (1996), Al-Saleh and Al-Khadari (2000), Barabasi-El-Shamawi (2001), Bouza (2002b), Chen (2001a, b), Yu-Lam (1997). A huge amount of papers are dedicated to the study of RSS as an alternative to the use of SRSWR, see for example Bai-Chen (2003), Muttlak-McDonald. (1992), and Chen-Bai (2001a). Different papers present a discussion of the State of the Art in RSS. We have the superb book on the theme Chen-Bai-Sinha (2004). It presents statistical inferences based on RSS and several experiments. Different recent oeuvres deal with discussions on certain aspects of the development of RSS, see for example Ahmad et al. (2010), where several authors present interesting issues on the theme from their perspective and experience.

The applications of RSS are not so widespread but since its beginnings applications was the motivation of developing the theory. Some of them are the estimation of mass herbage in a paddock, McIntyre (1978), Cobby et al.(1985), forage yields Halls-Dell (1966), and shrub Phytomass, Martin et al.(1980) and Muttlak-McDonald (1992), vegetation research Johnson et al. (1993), fishering Hankin-Reeves (1988), medicine as Chen-Stasny-Wolfe (2000): Some other results on the use of RSS in estimating plutonium soil concentrations are Gilbert (1995), in quality testing of reformulated gasoline as well as other technical issues as Nussbaum-Sinha (1997), and Al-Saleh-AL-Shrafat (2001).

When we deal with practical survey sampling the existence of missing observations is a usual problem to be solved. This oeuvre is concerned with the dealing with this problem in RSS applications and with the use or Randomized Responses for obtaining reliable information on sensitive variables.

To follow the ideas and proofs involved in RSS a knowledge of non-parametric statistics and sampling is needed at a level which is covered by advanced text books as Arnold et al. (1992), Sinha–Sinha-Purkayasthra (1996) and Hedayat-

Sinha (1992). A recent result is given in Arnold et al. (2009), where multivariate order statistics are considered in terms of their use in RSS:

The usual frame used in sampling theory considers a population and a variable of interest Y. A sampling design $d(s)$ is used for selecting a random sample s. The inclusion probabilities $\pi_i = \text{Prob}\,(u_i \in s)$ and $\pi_{ij} = \text{Prob}\,(u_i \wedge u_j \in s)$ are perfectly calculable. Once s is selected Y is evaluated on the sampled units and $y_1,...,y_n$ are obtained. A well-known estimator of the population mean μ is Horvitz-Thomson estimator $\mu_{HT} = \sum_{i \in s} Y_i / N\pi_i$. If SRS is used $\pi_i = n/N$ and μ_{HT} is the sample mean μ_s. Note that if we rank the observation and define the order statistics (os) $Y_{(i)}$, $i = 1,...,n$ we have $\mu_s = \frac{\sum_{i=1}^{n} Y_{(i)}}{n} = \mu_{(s)}$.

$$E(\mu_{(s)}) = \frac{\sum_{i=1}^{n} E(Y_{(i)})}{n} = \frac{\sum_{i=1}^{n} \mu_{(i)}}{n} = \mu.$$

When srswr is used the usual estimator of the population mean based on the observations is $\mu_s = \frac{\sum_{i=1}^{n} Y_i}{n}$. Its variance is $V(\mu_s) = \frac{\sum_{i=1}^{n} V(Y_i)}{n} = \frac{\sigma^2}{n}$.

If we base our inferences on the os's

$$V(\mu_{(s)}) = \frac{\sum_{i=1}^{n} V(Y_{(i)})}{n^2} = \frac{\sum_{i=1}^{n} \sigma_{(i)}^2}{n^2}$$

Note that the ranks do not intervene in the selection of the sample. We can define a map $g(u_i)$ such that it assigns to each sampled unit u_i a rank and only one. Each sampled unit may be ranked using g without measuring Y using some judgements. Say that the rank represents certain judgment on the value of Y. For example if we plan to study the stature of children we are able to rank them visually before selecting the sample. Similarly occurs when we use satellite information on the biomass for ecological studies. The first arising question is whether this ranking affects the behavior of a statistical procedure based in it. The first results in this theme considered that the rank was perfect, see McIntyre (1952), Takahasi-Wakimoto (1968). Dell-Clutter (1972) studied this problem considering a cumulative distribution function (cdf) p(y) in each sample unit were measured Y_i and *Rank [$Y_{(i)}$]*. Taking

$Y_{(i)} = i$-th judgment rank of the order statistics and $f_{(i)}$ (y) as its probability density function (pdf) we have that, as g is a one-to-one map $P(y) = \sum_{i=1}^{n} f_{(i)}(y)/n$ and $E[Y_{(i)}] = \sum_{t=1}^{n} Y_t f_{(y)}(y)/n = \mu_{(i)}$. Hence, when we deal with $\mu_{(s)}$ the unbiasedness property is maintained even using judgments and not the values of Y makes the ranking. Therefore,

$$\sum_{i=1}^{n} (\mu_{(i)} - \mu) = \sum_{i=1}^{n} \Delta_{(i)} = 0$$

The differences between the expected mean of the os's and the population mean play and important role in RSS because $\sigma_{(i)}^2 = \sigma^2 - \Delta_{(i)}^2$. Then

$$V[\mu_{(s)}] = \sum_{i=1}^{n} \sigma_{(i)}^2/n^2 = V[\mu_s] - \sum_{i=1}^{n} \Delta_{(i)}^2/n^2$$

Note that as $|\Delta_{(i)}|/\sigma \leq [\beta(2i-1, 2n-2i+1) - (\beta(i, n-i+1))^2]^{1/2}/(\beta(i, n-i+1))$

$$\sigma^2 \geq \Delta_{(i)}^2 (\beta(2i-1, 2n-2i+1))^2/[\beta(2i-1, 2n-2i+1) - (\beta(i, n-i+1))^2].$$

An extreme case is that in which none of the ranks assigned by judgement coincide with the true ones. The orders are considered as assigned by a random mechanism. Then $\Delta_{(i)} = 0$ for any $i = 1, \ldots, n$ and the RSS design is equivalent to the srs design. Patil et al. (1997a) discussed the notion of coherent sampling. Taking into account that we are sampling a set of units and that any sample s is a subset of the population $U;$ we can establish the following definition.

Definition 2.1 Define a protocol (a one-to-one map) g, which orders the units in a finite population $U(g(u_i) = \text{rank}(u_i))$ and induces an ordering on each $s \subset U$. It is called coherent if for any s and U the ranking induced on s is the same that the application of it directly in $s[g(u_i|U) < g(u_j|U) \Rightarrow (u_i|s) < g(u_j|s), \forall s \subset U, \forall i \neq j]$.

We consider the use of coherent ordering protocols. It allows using a global ranking of the units for ordering the observed sample without inconsistencies. Hence census information permits to establish an ordering in the sampled units. As pointed out by Patil et. al. (Patil et al. 1997a) if we have a coherent RSS design we are implementing an imperfect stratification. The knowledge of the true ranks of all the population units allows using them for stratifying. Some kind of optimal stratification can be implemented and it will provide more accurate estimates than RSS. Therefore, g permits to stratify in 'small sets' where each member have very similar values of Y.

We may rank using judgments. It can be characterized by an auxiliary variable X related with Y. David-Levine (1972) quoted this problem. Dell-Clutter (1972) analyzed the case in which the ranking is made with errors and established that the usual estimates from the computed os's maintain the unbiasedness property. Stokes (1977a, b) used this result by considering that X is known for any unit and is used for ranking. An apparent source of errors in RSS is the use of X for ranking. A practical methodology is to consider that we select s and the sequence $X_{(1)}, \ldots, X_{(n)}$ is obtained.

Take the location model $Y_{(i)} = X_{(i)} + e_i, i = 1, \ldots, n$ and consider that the random errors have null expectation $[E(e_i) = 0, i = 1, \ldots, n]$. A common assumption is that they are independently normal variables with variance σ_i^2. It is clear that the RSS estimator is still unbiased.

Another model is to consider that the regression $Y_i = a + bX_i + e_i, i = 1, \ldots, n$ characterizes the relationship between two equally distributed variables X and Y.

The correct os is $Y_{(i)}$ but as the regression allows to fix that $E\left[Y_{(i)}|X_{(i)}\right] = \mu_Y + \rho\sigma_Y[X_{(i)} - \mu_X]/\sigma_X], i = 1, \ldots, n$ and then, if X and Y are positively correlated the os determined by X and by Y will be the similar.

2.2 The Basic RSS Strategy

2.2.1 The Sampling Procedure

The theoretical frame that permits to use the RSS model is based on the hypothesis:

i.   We wish to enumerate the measurable variable Y.
ii.   The units can be ordered linearly without ties.
iii. Any sample $s \subset U$ of size m can be enumerated.
iv.   To identify a unit, order the units in s and enumerate them which is less costly than to evaluate $\{Y_i, i \in s\}$ or to order U.

The first hypothesis is commonly assumed in the general theory of sampling problem, the second fixes that the rank can be made without confusions and that any rank is assigned to only one of the sampled units. The third assumption is also common in the applications. The fourth has an economical and a statistical motivation: only if it is cheap to rank RSS is a good alternative with respect to rank all the units of U and to stratify, which is more accurate. Some definitions are needed.

Definition 2.2 A statistical sampling unit (ssu) is a set s with m units of U.
Usually m ssu's are selected independently.

In survey sampling settings, it is logic rankingof the units based on the values of an auxiliary variable correlated with the variable of interest. The basic RSS procedure is the following:

Step 1:   Randomly select m^2 units from the target population. These units are randomly allocated into m sets, each of size m.
Step 2:   The m units of each set are ranked visually or by any inexpensive method free of cost, say X, with respect to the variable of interest Y. From the first set of m units, the smallest ranked unit is measured; from the second set of m units the second smallest ranked unit is measured. Continue until the mth smallest unit (the largest) is measured from the last set.
Step 3:   Repeat the whole process $r(i)$ times (cycles).
Step 4:   Evaluate the corresponding units.

We can denote it as follows

$$
\left.\begin{array}{c} X_{i1} \\ X_{i2} \\ \vdots \\ X_{im} \end{array}\right\}_{r} \sim > X_{(ii)r} = Y_{(i)r}, r = 1, \ldots, r(i); i = 1, \ldots, m
$$

Let $Y_1, \ldots, Y_m$ be a sample selected using SRSWR from probability density function $f(y)$, with mean μ_Y and variance σ_Y^2. Considering the selection of m independent samples selected using a SRSWR design, of size m each, we have $Y_{11}, \ldots, Y_{1m}, Y_{21}, \ldots, Y_{2m}, \ldots .Y_{m1}, \ldots, Y_{mm}$. Let $Y_{i(1m)}, \ldots, Y_{i(mm)}, \ldots Y_{i(mm)}$, be the order statistics of the sample $Y_{1i}, \ldots, Y_{1m}, , \ldots, Y_{im}$, for $(i = 1, 2, \ldots, m)$.

Takahasi and Wakimoto (1968) provided the mathematical theory of RSS and showed that $f(y) = \frac{\sum_{j=1}^m f_{(jm)}(y)}{m}$, $\mu_Y = \frac{\sum_{j=1}^m \mu_{Y_{(jm)}}(y)}{m}$ and $V(Y_{(jm)} = \sigma_{Y_{(jm)}}^2 - \Delta_{Y_{(jm)}}^2$, $\Delta_{Y_{(jm)}}^2 = \left(\mu_{Y_{(jm)}} - \mu_Y\right)^2, j = 1, \ldots, m$.

Without losing in generality we will drop the value m of the sample size in the notation in the sequel when it provides no further information.

Note that if $r = 1$ we observe only a RSS of size $m = n$.

Definition 2.3 When $r(i) = r$ the RSS design is denominated as balanced and unbalanced otherwise.

For balanced RSS designs, we have that each sample $s(j)$ is a SRSWR of size r and $n = rm$.

2.2.2 Estimation of μ

The usual estimator of μ_Z, for a variable Z, is $\mu_{Z(\text{rss})} = \frac{\sum_{j=1}^m \sum_{i=1}^r Z_{(i:i)j}}{n}, n = rm$.

Noting that for any j, $E\left(Z_{(i:i)j}\right) = \mu_{Z_{(i)}}$ the unbiasedness of this estimator is easily derived because

$$
E(\mu_{Z(\text{rss})}) = \frac{\sum_{j=1}^m \sum_{i=1}^r \mu_{Z_{(i)}}}{n} = \frac{\sum_{j=1}^m \mu_{Z_{(i)}}}{m} = \mu_Z
$$

The samples $s(j)$ are independent. Hence, the variance of $\mu_{Z(\text{rss})}$ is:

$$
V\left(\mu_{Z(\text{rss})}\right) = \frac{\sum_{j=1}^m \sum_{i=1}^r \sigma_{Z(i)}^2}{n^2} = \frac{\sum_{j=1}^m \sigma_{Z(i)}^2}{rm^2} = \frac{\sigma_Z^2}{n} - \frac{\sum_{j=1}^m \Delta_{Y_{(jm)}}^2}{mn},
$$

$$
\Delta_{Y_{(jm)}}^2 = \left(\mu_{Z_{(j)}} - \mu_Z\right)^2, \ n = rm.
$$

This allows writing

$$\sigma_Z^2 = \frac{\left(\sum_{i=1}^r \sigma_{Z_{(i)}}^2 + \sum_{i=1}^r \mu_{Z_{(i)}}^2 - \mu_Z^2\right)}{r}$$

Note that once we know that m is fixed, the notation may be simplified dropping the subscript m and writing $Y_{(j:t)}$ for denoting the jth-os of the t-th ranked sample $s(t)$.

Definition 2.4 The relative precision of μ_{RSS} with respect to μ_s is $RP(\mu_s, \mu_{\mathrm{rss}}) = \frac{V(\mu_{\mathrm{srs}})}{V(\mu_{\mathrm{rss}})}$ and the relative saving (RS) due to RSS is measured by $RS = 1 - \frac{1}{RP}$. □

The net gain in accuracy due to the use of RSS is measured by $\frac{\sum_{j=1}^m \Delta_{Y_{(j:j)}}^2}{mn}$.

In the balanced case $RP \in [1, (m+1)/2]$ and in the unbalanced $RP \in [1, m]$. The later depends on the allocation of the sample. Patil et al. (1997b) established that if we deal with a skewed distribution or if an adequate stratification is implemented the unbalanced design may not be so efficient. RS may be used with the purpose of evaluating the relative gain in accuracy due to the use of RSS.

Kaur et al. (1996) studied the allocation problem. When Neymann's allocation principle is used for determining $r(i)$'s and n is fixed the optimal sample sizes are given by:

$$r^*(i) = \frac{n\sigma_{Y_{(i)}}^2}{\sum_{j=1}^m \sigma_{Y_{(j)}}^2}$$

Another approach is based on the knowledge of the existence of a large tail pdf. In the case of a heavy right tail, a skewed distribution we have that the os's variance are ordered and $\sigma_{(1)}^2 \le \sigma_{(2)}^2 \le \cdots \le \sigma_{(m)}^2$. The statistician fixes a constant $\theta > 1$ and $r^* \equiv r(i) = r(m)/\theta$, $i = 1, \ldots, m-1$. Then

$$V(\mu_{\mathrm{rss}}|\theta) = \frac{\sum_{j=1}^{m-1} \frac{\sigma_{Y_{(j)}}^2}{r^*} + \frac{\sigma_{Y_{(m)}}^2}{\theta r^*}}{m^2}$$

Hence, using a larger number of replicas reduces seriously the summand with larger variance of the os.

The use of $r > 1$ is justified by practical reasons mainly. To rank subjectively the units are easier when m is small. Hence for obtaining a sample of size n is better to repeat the selection or m^2 RSS samples r times once $n = rm$. Some evidence on the usefulness of the usage of small m and large r is present in studies with particular distributions.

Usually, SRSWR is used for selecting the samples independently but simple random sampling without replacement may be used (SRSWOR). This is more important when we study a finite population because a correction should be introduced for computing the sampling error. The problem is certainly very complicated when compared with the usual one. Patil et al. (1995) derived the expression of the corresponding variance. A gain in precision due to RSS now depends heavily on the replication factor. The theoretical problems associated with the use of os in finite population sampling using RSS are the kernel of the behavior of the wor procedure. Lehman (1966) established some properties of the random variables generated by a univariate distribution and their os's. One of them is that any pair of os's has a joint pdf, which is positively likelihood ratio dependent. Then, if we sample a finite population of os's using srswor this property holds. Takasi-Fututsya (1998) used these results for deriving a method for computing the finite population correction factor.

2.2.3 The Estimation of the Variance

Let us consider the estimation of the variance. For details see Stokes (1977a, b, 1980) and Yanagawa (2000). An unbiased estimator of $\sigma^2_{Y_{(j)}}$ is

$$\hat{\sigma}^2_{Z_{(i)}} = \frac{\sum_{j=1}^{r}\left(Z_{(i:m)j} - \hat{\mu}_{Z_{(i:m)}}\right)^2}{r-1}, \quad \hat{\mu}_{Z_{(i:m)}} = \frac{\sum_{j=1}^{r} Z_{(i:m)j}}{r}, i = 1,\ldots,m$$

Hence, an unbiased estimator of the variance $\sigma^2_Z = \frac{\sum_{j=1}^{N}(Z_j - \mu_Z)^2}{N}, \mu_Z = \frac{\sum_{j=1}^{N} Z_j}{N}$ using RSS is

$$\hat{\sigma}^2_Z = \frac{(n-m+1)\sum_{j=1}^{m}\sum_{i=1}^{r}\left(Z_{(i:m)j} - \hat{\mu}_{Z_{(i:m)}}\right)^2}{n\,r(r-1)} + \frac{\sum_{j=1}^{r}\left(\hat{\mu}_{Z_{(i:m)}} - \mu_{Z(\mathrm{rss})}\right)^2}{m}, \hat{\mu}_{Z_{(i:m)}}$$

$$= \frac{\sum_{j=1}^{m} Z_{(i:m)j}}{r}$$

An analysis establishes that the first term is the "within" variation and the second one means from the "between" variation source in terms of the cycles. Note that it cannot be used when $r = 1$.

Stokes (1980) considered the use of the naïve estimator

$$\hat{\sigma}^2_{Z(\mathrm{rss})} = \frac{\sum_{j=1}^{m}\sum_{i=1}^{r}\left(Z_{(i:m)j} - \hat{\mu}_{Z_{(\mathrm{rss})}}\right)^2}{n-1} = \frac{\sum_{i=1}^{n}\left(Z_{(ii)} - \mu_{Z(\mathrm{rss})}\right)^2}{n-1}$$

It is worthy to note that the naïve estimator of σ^2_Z can be used also for $r = 1$. It is not unbiased because

$$E(\hat{\sigma}^2_{Z\text{rss}}) = \frac{E\left(\sum_{i=1}^n Z^2_{(ii)}\right)}{n(n-1)} - \frac{\sum_{i \neq j=1}^n E(Z_{(ii)})E(Z_{(jj)})}{n}$$

$$> \frac{E\left(\sum_{i=1}^n Z^2_{(ii)}\right)}{n(n-1)} - \frac{\sum_{i \neq j=1}^n E(Z_{(ii)}Z_{(jj)})}{n} = \sigma^2_Z$$

$$\hat{\sigma}^2_{Z(m,r)} = \frac{\sum_{j=1}^m \sum_{i=1}^r \left(Z_{(i:m)j} - \hat{\mu}_{Z_{(rss)}}\right)^2}{n-1}$$

It is asymptotically unbiased because

$$E(\hat{\sigma}^2_{Z(m,r)}) = \sigma^2_Z + \frac{\sum_{j=1}^m \sum_{i=1}^r \left(\mu_{Z\,(i:m)} - \mu_Z\right)^2}{m(n-1)}$$

and $\frac{\sum_{j=1}^m \sum_{i=1}^r \left(\mu_{Z\,(i:m)} - \mu_Z\right)^2}{m(n-1)} \to 0$ for m or r large.

The relative precision of this estimator is

$$RP\left(\sigma^2_Z, \sigma^2_{Z(m,r)}\right) = \frac{V(\hat{\sigma}^2_Z)}{MSE(\hat{\sigma}^2_{Z(m,r)})} = \frac{V(\hat{\sigma}^2_Z)}{V\left(\hat{\sigma}^2_{Z(m,r)}\right) + \left(\frac{\sum_{i=1}^r \left(\mu_{Z\,(i:m)} - \mu_Z\right)^2}{m(n-1)}\right)^2}$$

where $\hat{\sigma}^2_Z = \frac{\sum_{j=1}^n (Z_i - \bar{Z})^2}{n-1}, \bar{Z} = \frac{\sum_{j=1}^n Z_i}{n}$. It is worthy to note that $\frac{\sum_{i=1}^r \left(\mu_{Z\,(i:m)} - \mu_Z\right)^2}{m(n-1)}$ is a decreasing function of m and r and $\frac{\sum_{i=1}^r \left(\mu_{Z\,(i:m)} - \mu_Z\right)^2}{m} < \sigma^2_Z$. As a consequence $\left(\hat{\sigma}^2_Z, \hat{\sigma}^2_{Z(m,r)}\right) < \text{ARE}\left(\hat{\sigma}^2_Z, \hat{\sigma}^2_{m,r}\right)$. Hence, this estimator is used frequently in statistical inferences because $\lim_{k \to \infty} RP\left(\hat{\sigma}^2_Z, \hat{\sigma}^2_{Z(m,r)}\right) = ARE\left(\hat{\sigma}^2_Z, \hat{\sigma}^2_{Z(m,r)}\right), k = m \text{ or } r$.

In practice m is small, for ranking adequately and cheaply, but we are able to fix a large number of cycles.

Therefore, the relative precisions can be estimated using the ratio between the estimated variance.

2.2.4 Confidence Intervals

The estimators (averages across de sets)

$$\mu^*_{Z_{(j)}} = \frac{\sum_{i=1}^m Z_{(i:m)j}}{m}, j = 1, \ldots, r$$

are independent and identically distributed (iid) with expectation μ_Z. Their variances are proportional to $\sum_{i=1}^{m} \sigma_{Z_{(i)}}^2$.

An estimator of $\sigma_{Z_{(i)}}^2$, the variance across cycles, is

$$\hat{\sigma}_{Z_{(i)}}^{*2} = \frac{\sum_{j=1}^{r} \left(Z_{(i:m)j} - \hat{\mu}_{Z_{(i:m)}} \right)^2}{r-1}$$

It is consistent because it is the variance of iid variables and as a consequence $\sum_{i=1}^{m} \hat{\sigma}_{Z_{(i)}}^2$ is consistent for $V(\mu_{Z_{(j)}}^*)$ which is proportional to $\sum_{i=1}^{m} \sigma_{Z_{(i)}}^2$.

Approximate confidence intervals can be derived, using the consistency of the estimators, using the fact that $m\sqrt{r} \left(\frac{\mu_{Z_{rss}} - \mu_Z}{\sqrt{\sum_{i=1}^{m} \hat{\sigma}_{Z_{(i)}}^2}} \right) \to_d N(0,1)$.

For further reading is recommended Chen et al. (2004).

2.3 Some Other RSS Strategies

Some transformations to the basic RSS design have been proposed. We will present some of the most popular for finite population framework. They use some criteria that are good for certain particular cases in terms of their accuracy, measured in terms of the variance. We will present them for one cycle. The development for $r > 1$ is straightforward.

2.3.1 Median RSS Sampling (MRSS)

The MRSS procedure was proposed by Muttlak (1995). Muttlak (1998 and 2003) proposed to select the median of $s(j)$ in each ssu. The pdf of Y must have finite mean and variances μ and σ^2. We observe $\left\{ Y_{(1:1)}, ..., Y_{(1:m)}, Y_{(2:1)}, ..., Y_{(m:m)} \right\}_t$, $t = 1, ..., r$. If m is odd the os's measured are $Y_{(j:med)t}^* = Y_{\left(\frac{m+1}{2}:m\right)t}$, $t = 1, .., r$. If m is even is used

$$Y_{(j:med)t}^* = \begin{cases} Y_{\left(\frac{m}{2}:m\right)t} & \text{if } m < \frac{m}{2} + 1 \\ Y_{\left(\frac{m}{2}+1:m\right)t} & \text{if } m > \frac{m}{2}, \end{cases}$$

$$t = 1, \ldots, r$$

The estimator is $\mu_{\mathrm{rss[med]}} = \frac{\sum_{j=1}^{m}\sum_{t=1}^{r} Y^{*}_{(j:\mathrm{med})t}}{mr}$ and its expectation is

$E\left(\mu_{\mathrm{rss[med]}}\right) = \frac{\sum_{j=1}^{m}\mu_{Y\,(j:\mathrm{med})}}{m}$. Note that for n odd $\mu_{Y\,(j:\mathrm{med})} = \mu_{Y\,(\frac{m+1}{2})}$ for any j, then

$E\left(\mu_{\mathrm{rss[med]}}\right) = \mu_{Y(\frac{m+1}{2})}$. If m is even $E\left(\mu_{Y\,\mathrm{rss[med]}}\right) = \frac{\mu_{Y}\left(\frac{m}{2}\right)+\mu_{Y}\left(\frac{m}{2}+1\right)}{2}$.

The variance of the estimator is given by

$$V\left(\mu_{Y\,\mathrm{rss[med]}}\right) = \frac{\sum_{j=1}^{m}\sigma^{2}_{Y\,(j:\mathrm{med})}}{m^{2}r} = \frac{\sigma^{2}_{Y}}{n} - \frac{\sum_{j=1}^{m}\Delta^{2}_{Y\,(j:\mathrm{med})}}{mn}$$

where

$$\Delta^{2}_{Y\,(j:\mathrm{med})} = \begin{cases} \left(\mu_{Y\,(\frac{m+1}{2})} - \mu_{Y}\right)^{2} & \text{if } m \text{ is odd} \\[2mm] \left(\mu_{Y\,(\frac{m}{2})} - \mu_{Y}\right)^{2} & \text{if } m \text{ is even and } j \le \frac{m}{2} \\[2mm] \left(\mu_{Y\,(\frac{m}{2}+1)} - \mu_{Y}\right)^{2} & \text{if } m \text{ is even and } j > \frac{m}{2} \end{cases}$$

Muttlak's estimator is unbiased only if the pdf is symmetric with respect to μ and $V\left(\mu_{Y\,\mathrm{rss[med]}}\right) \le V(\mu_{Y\,\mathrm{rss}}) \le V(\mu_{Y\,s})$. The relative precision of it (RP) increases with m. For not symmetric pdf's the estimator is still more precise than the arithmetic mean of SRS, $\mu_{Y\,s}$, but it is biased. The RP decreases if $m \ge 6$. The errors in the ranking do not affect seriously these results. Hence the use of median-RSS provides a gain in accuracy.

2.3.2 Extreme RSS Sampling (ERSS)

Another particular procedure is to use the extreme os of the samples. Further reading can be obtained in Samawi et al. (1996), Bhoj (1997). That is, in each RSS sample we measure $Y_{(1:j)}$ and $Y_{(n:j)}$. Take m even and compute

$$Y_{(j:e)} = \frac{Y_{(1:j)} + Y_{(m:j)}}{2}$$

Its expectation and variances are, as SRSWR is used,

$$E\left(Y_{(j:e)}\right) = \frac{\mu_{Y\,(1)} + \mu_{Y\,(m)}}{2}, \quad V\left(Y_{(j:e)}\right) = \frac{\sigma^{2}_{Y\,(1)} + \sigma^{2}_{Y\,(m)}}{4}$$

Samawi et al. (1996) proposed the estimator:

$$\mu_{Y\,\mathrm{rss}(e)} = \frac{\sum_{j=1}^{m} Y_{(j:e)}}{m}$$

This estimator also is biased because

$$E\left(\mu_{Y\ \mathrm{rss}(e)}\right) = \frac{\mu_{Y\ (1)} + \mu_{Y\ (m)}}{2}$$

and

$$V\left(\mu_{Y\ \mathrm{rss}(e)}\right) = \frac{\sigma_{Y\ (1)}^2 + \sigma_{Y(m)}^2}{2m}$$

For m odd the variable used is

$$Y_{(j:e)}^* = \begin{cases} Y_{(1:j)} & \text{if } j < m \text{ and } j \text{ odd} \\ Y_{(m:j)} & \text{if } j < m \text{ and } j \text{ even} \\ \dfrac{Y_{(1:j)} + Y_{(m:j)}}{2} & \text{if } j = m \end{cases}$$

An estimator of the population mean is $\mu_{\mathrm{rss}(e)}^* = \frac{\sum_{j=1}^{m} Y_{(j:e)}^*}{m}$.
Its expectation is equal to the expectation of $\mu_{RSS[e]}$ but

$$V\left(\mu_{\mathrm{rss}(e)}^*\right) = \frac{\sigma_{Y\ (1,m)}}{2m^2} + \frac{(2m-1)\left(\sigma_{Y\ (1)}^2 + \sigma_{Y\ (m)}^2\right)}{4m^2},$$

$$\sigma_{Y\ (1,m)} = \mathrm{Cov}(Y_{(1:m)}, Y_{m:m})$$

An alternative estimator analyzed for m odd is:

$$\mu_{\mathrm{rss}(e)}^{**} = \frac{\sum_{j=1}^{m-1} Y_{(j:e)} + Y_{\left(\frac{m+1}{2}:m\right)}}{m}$$

It is also biased as

$$E\left(\mu_{\mathrm{rss}(e)}^{**}\right) = \frac{(m+1)\left(\mu_{Y\ (1)} + \mu_{Y\ (n)}\right)}{2m} + \frac{\mu_{Y\ \left(\frac{m+1}{2}\right)}}{m}$$

which variance is:

$$V\left(\mu_{\mathrm{rss}(e)}^{**}\right) = \frac{\sigma_{Y\ \left(\frac{m+1}{2}\right)}^2}{m^2} + \frac{(m-1)\left(\sigma_{Y\ (1)}^2 + \sigma_{Y(n)}^2\right)}{2m^2}$$

If the pdf is symmetric with respect to $\mu_Y = 0$ the median is equal to zero. From the results of Arnold et al. (1992) we have that, in this case:

1. $\mu_{Y\ (1)} = -\mu_{Y\ (n)}$ for m even and $\mu_{(\lfloor m+1 \rfloor/2)} = 0$ if m is odd.
2. $\sigma_{Y\ (1)}^2 = \sigma_{Y\ (n)}^2$

Therefore in this particular case:

$$E\left(\mu_{rss(e)}\right) = E\left(\mu^*_{rss(e)}\right) = E\left(\mu^{**}_{rss(e)}\right) = 0$$

$$V\left(\mu_{rss(e)}\right) = \frac{\sigma^2_{Y\,(1)}}{m}, V\left(\mu^*_{rss(e)}\right) = \frac{(2m-1)\left(\sigma^2_{Y\,(1)} + \sigma_{Y\,(1,n)}\right)}{2m^2},$$

$$V\left(\mu^{**}_{rss(e)}\right) = \frac{(m-1)\left(\sigma^2_{Y\,(1)} + \sigma^2_{Y\,(1)\left(\frac{m+1}{2}\right)}\right)}{m^2}$$

When the distribution is uniform these estimators have a smaller variance than μ_s. The preference of one or another estimator depends of the value of m including when compared with the use of the usual RSS estimator.

2.3.3   L-RSS Sampling

The L-RSS procedure is described, following the paper of Al-Nasser (2007). It is implemented by the following procedure.

2.3.3.1   L-RSS Procedure

Step 1: Randomly select m^2 units from the target population of size N, ($U = \{1, \ldots, N\}$.

Step 2:   Rank the units within each set with respect to the variable of interest Y

Step 3:   Calculate $k = [mp]$, $p \in [0, 1/2]$.

Step 4:   For $i \leq k$ select the units with rank $k + 1$.

Step 5:   For $k < i \leq m-k-1$ measure the units with rank i.

Step 6:   For each $i \geq m-k$ measure the unit with rank $m-k$.

Step 7:   Repeat the steps $1-6$ r times.

The estimator proposed by Al-Nasser (2007), when $r = 1$, $m = n$ and is

$$\bar{y}_{\text{LRSS}} = \frac{\sum_{i=1}^{k} Y_{i(k+1)} + \sum_{i=k+1}^{n-k} Y_{i(i)} + \sum_{i=n-k+1}^{n} Y_{i(n-k)}}{m}$$

Its variance is given by

$$V(\bar{y}_{\text{LRSS}}) = \frac{\sum_{i=1}^{k} V(Y_{i(k+1)}) + \sum_{i=k+1}^{n-k} V(Y_{i(i)}) + \sum_{i=n-k+1}^{n} V(Y_{i(n-k)})}{n^2}$$

Remembering that the expectation of an os is

$$E(Y_{i(j)}) = \mu_{Y_{(j)}} = \mu_Y + (\mu_{\mu_{Y_{(j)}}} - \mu_Y) = \mu_Y + \Delta_{Y\,(j)}$$

we have that

$$nE(\bar{y}_{\text{LRSS}}) = k[\mu_{Y\,(k+1)} + \mu_{Y\,(n-k+1)}] + \sum_{i=k+1}^{n-k} \mu_{Y\,(i)}$$

$$= \mu_Y + k[\Delta_{Y\,(k+1)} + \Delta_{Y\,(m-k)}] + \sum_{i=k+1}^{n-k} \Delta_{Y\,(i)}$$

Therefore, when the distribution is symmetric this estimator is unbiased. Taking into account that the variance of an order statistics is $(Y_{i(j)}) = \sigma_{Y_{(j)}}^2 = \sigma_Y^2 - \Delta_{Y\,(j)}^2$. We have that

$$V(\bar{y}_{\text{LRSS}}) = \frac{kr[\sigma_{Y_{(k+1)}}^2 + \sigma_{Y\,(n-k-1)}^2] + r\sum_{i=k+1}^{n-k} \sigma_{Y_{(i)}}^2}{n^2}$$

2.4 Some Particular Estimators

2.4.1 The Ratio Estimator

2.4.1.1 Usual Estimator

One of the most popular estimation problems is to estimate the ratio. Consider as usual that X is well known and that it is used for ranking. The selection of a sample of size n yields the estimators based on a RSS-same are

$$\bar{y}_{\text{rss}} = \frac{\sum_{i=1}^{n} y_{(i:i)}}{n}, \quad \bar{x}_{rss} = \frac{\sum_{i=1}^{n} x_{(i:i)}}{n}$$

The ratio estimator of the mean is

$$\bar{y}_{r-\text{rss}} = \frac{\bar{y}_{\text{rss}}}{\bar{x}_{\text{rss}}} \mu_X$$

Its study is developed using some expansion in Taylor Series $E(\bar{y}_{r-\text{rss}} - \mu_Y)^2$. Using it is obtained that the MSE is given by:

$$M(\bar{y}_{r-\text{rss}}) = \frac{\sigma_y^2 - \sum_{i=1}^{m}\frac{\Delta_{Y(i)}^2}{m} + R^2\left[\sigma_x^2 - \sum_{i=1}^{m}\frac{\Delta_{X(i)}^2}{m}\right] - 2R\rho\left(\sigma_x^2 - \sum_{i=1}^{m}\frac{\Delta_{X(i)}^2}{m}\right)^{1/2} x \left(\sigma_y^2 - \sum_{i=1}^{m}\frac{\Delta_{Y(i)}^2}{m}\right)^{1/2}}{n}$$

Then we prefer this estimator to the SRSWR one when

$$\delta_{r-\text{rss}} = \frac{\sum_{i=1}^{m}\frac{\Delta_{Y(i)}^2}{m} + R^2\sum_{i=1}^{m}\frac{\Delta_{Y(i)}^2}{m} - 2R\rho\left[\sigma_X\sigma_Y - \left(\sigma_x^2 - \sum_{i=1}^{m}\frac{\Delta_{X(i)}^2}{m}\right)^{1/2} x \left(\sigma_y^2 - \sum_{i=1}^{m}\frac{\Delta_{Y(i)}^2}{m}\right)^{1/2}\right]}{n} > 0$$

In terms of the correlation we have that RSS should be preferred to SRSWR estimator if

$$\rho < \frac{\sum_{i=1}^{m}\frac{\Delta_{Y(i)}^2}{m} + R^2\sum_{i=1}^{m}\frac{\Delta_{Y(i)}^2}{m}}{2R\left[\sigma_X\sigma_Y - \sqrt{\left(\sigma_x^2 - \sum_{i=1}^{m}\frac{\Delta_{X(i)}^2}{m}\right)} x \sqrt{\left(\sigma_y^2 - \sum_{i=1}^{m}\frac{\Delta_{Y(i)}^2}{m}\right)}\right]}$$

The terms under the square root sign are positive, as they are variances. Then, we can rewrite the relationship deriving that

$$\rho < \frac{\sum_{i=1}^{m}\frac{\Delta_{Y(i)}^2}{m} + R^2\sum_{i=1}^{m}\frac{\Delta_{Y(i)}^2}{m}}{2R\left[\sigma_X\sigma_Y\left(1 - \left(1 - \sum_{i=1}^{m}\frac{\Delta_{X(i)}^2}{m\sigma_x^2}\right)^{1/2}\left(1 - \sum_{i=1}^{m}\frac{\Delta_{Y(i)}^2}{m\sigma_y^2}\right)^{1/2}\right)\right]}$$

The right-hand side of the equation is positive then, if $\rho < 0$, RSS is better than SRSWR strategy.

Take $r > 1$ and note that X is known then we can compute the mean of the $rm^2 = mn$ selected units

$$\bar{\bar{x}} = \frac{\sum_{t=1}^{r}\sum_{i=1}^{m}\sum_{j-1}^{m}x_{(i,j)t}}{rm^2}$$

Therefore, we may use another ratio estimator defined as

$$\bar{y}_{r-\text{rss}2} = \bar{y}_{(0,1,0)-\text{rss}2} = \frac{\bar{y}_{\text{rss}}}{\bar{\bar{x}}}\overline{X}$$

We use *rss2* to distinguish this proposal from $\bar{y}_{r-rss}$, and

$$M(\bar{y}_{r-\text{rsss2}}) = \frac{\sigma_y^2 - \sum_{i=1}^{m}\frac{\Delta_{Y(i)}^2}{m} + R^2\frac{\sigma_x^2}{r} - 2R\rho\frac{\sigma_x}{\sqrt{r_x}}\left(\sigma_y^2 - \sum_{i=1}^{m}\frac{\Delta_{Y(i)}^2}{m}\right)^{1/2}}{n}$$

This estimator should be preferred to the classic ratio estimator when the following inequality holds

$$\delta_{r-\text{rsss2}} = \frac{\sum_{i=1}^{m}\frac{\Delta_{Y(i)}^2}{m} - 2R\rho\left[\frac{\sigma_X\sigma_Y}{\sqrt{r}} - \left(1 - \sum_{i=1}^{m}\frac{\Delta_{Y(i)}^2}{m\sigma_Y}\right)^{1/2}\right]}{n} > 0$$

That is if

$$\rho < \frac{\sum_{i=1}^{m}\frac{\Delta_{Y(i)}^2}{m}}{2R\left[\frac{\sigma_X\sigma_Y}{\sqrt{r}} - \left(1 - \sum_{i=1}^{m}\frac{\Delta_{Y(i)}^2}{m\sigma_Y}\right)^{1/2}\right]}$$

A comparison between the two RSS strategies determines that a preference for this estimator is a result when

$$M(\bar{y}_{r-\text{rss}}) - M(\bar{y}_{r-\text{rsss2}}) > 0$$

that is if

$$\delta_{\text{rss,rss2}} = \frac{R^2\sigma_X^2\left(1-\frac{1}{r}\right) - R^2\left[\sum_{i=1}^{m}\frac{\Delta_{X(i)}^2}{m}\right] - 2R\rho\sigma_X\left[\left(1 - \sum_{i=1}^{m}\frac{\Delta_{X(i)}^2}{m\sigma_X}\right)^{1/2} - \frac{1}{\sqrt{r}}\right]\left(\sigma_y^2 - \sum_{i=1}^{m}\frac{\Delta_{Y(i)}^2}{m}\right)^{1/2}}{n} > 0$$

It is biased but the bias usually is small with respect to *n*. Bouza (2001a, b) used RSS for selecting a sample using a third variable related with *X* and *Y*.

2.4.1.2 Median Ratio Estimator

The use of ratio-tupe estimators using RSS is receiving more attention from the researchers recently, see for example Al-Omari et al. (2008, 2009), Bouza and Al-Omari (2011a).

One of the first approaches of RSS for ratio estimation is due Samawi-Muttlak (1996). They assumed that the auxiliary variable *X* is ranked without error, $r = 1$. The observation $(X_{(i:j)t}, Y_{(i:j)t})$ is the pair of values in the i-th judgment os in the RSS sample *s(j)*. Their proposal was not to use the pairs in the diagonal but the medians

$$Z^*_{(i:j)} = \begin{cases} Z_{\left(\frac{n+1}{2}:j\right)} & \text{if } n \text{ is odd} \\ \dfrac{Z_{\left(\frac{n}{2}:j\right)} + Z_{\left(\frac{n+2}{2}:j\right)}}{2} & \text{if } n \text{ is even} \end{cases} \quad, Z = X, Y$$

The estimation of the mean is made by averaging the $Z^*_{(i:j)t}$'s.

$$\mu_{rss[m]Z^*} = \frac{\sum_{j=1}^{m} Z^*_{(i:j)}}{n}, Z = X, Y$$

The estimator of the ratio based on these RSS median-based estimators of the mean is $R_m = \frac{\mu_{rss[m]Y^*}}{\mu_{rss[m]X^*}}$. Taking

$$V_{Z_{(h)}} = \frac{\sigma^2_{Z_{(h)}}}{\mu^2_Z}, Z = X, Y, C_{(h)} = \frac{\mathrm{Cov}\left(X_{(h)}, Y_{(h)}\right)}{\mu_X \mu_Y}$$

The variance of this estimator is:

$$V(R_m) = \begin{cases} \dfrac{R^2 V_{X_{\left(\frac{n+1}{2}\right)}} + V_{Y_{\left(\frac{n+1}{2}\right)}} - C_{\left(\frac{n+1}{2}\right)}}{n} & \text{if } n \text{ is odd} \\ \dfrac{R^2 V_{X_{\left(\frac{n}{2}\right)}} + V_{Y_{\left(\frac{n}{2}\right)}} - 2\left(C_{\left(\frac{n}{2}\right)} + C_{\left(\frac{n+2}{2}\right)}\right)}{n} & \text{if } n \text{ is even} \end{cases}$$

The involved variances of the RSS estimators are expressed as the difference between a function of the population variance of Z and a function of sum of the $\Delta_i^{2'}s$. The relative merit of this strategy is that the estimation is fitted in a non-parametric sense and we need to rank only a part of the sample. Other intents in this line are presented in Patil et al. (1997a, b).

2.4.1.3 Ratio Estimator's Classes

A large class of ratio type estimators is given by fixing a vector of parameters $\theta = (\alpha, B, \lambda)^T$, where $\alpha \in A$, $B \in B*$, $\lambda \in L$. Denote this class as

$$F = \left\{ \bar{y}_\theta = \frac{\bar{Y}_{est} + \alpha}{B\bar{X}_{est} + \lambda}(B\bar{X} + \lambda); \theta = (\alpha, B, \lambda)^T \in A \times B^* \times L \right\}$$

$\bar{Z}_{est}$, $Z = X$, Y, is an estimator to the corresponding mean. Consider

$$\begin{aligned} A &= \{0, & b(\bar{X} - \bar{x}), & \sigma_x\} = \{\alpha_1, \alpha_2, \alpha_3\} \\ B^* &= \{1, & B_2(x), & C_x, & \rho\} = \{B_1, B_2, B_3.B_4\} \\ L &= \{0, & \rho, & B_2(x), & C_x\} = \{\lambda_1, \lambda_2, \lambda_3.\lambda_4\}. \end{aligned}$$

where

$b = s_{xy}/s_x^2$ is the linear regression coefficient
$B_2(x)$ is the coefficient of kurtosis of the distribution of X
C_x is the variation coefficient of X
ρ is the coefficient of linear correlation between X and Y

Then, this class contains some well-known estimators. For example, the classic estimator is obtained when $\theta = (0, 1, 0) = (\alpha_1, B_1, \lambda_1)$ as

$$\bar{y}_r = \bar{y}_{(0,1,0)} = \frac{\bar{y}}{\bar{x}} \overline{X}$$

The mean squared error of the corresponding subclass is characterized by
$M(\bar{y}_{razn}) = \frac{\sigma_y^2 + R^2 \sigma_x^2 w(w - 2\gamma)}{n}$ with $w = 1$, $\gamma = \rho \frac{C_y}{C_x} = \rho \frac{\frac{\sigma_y}{\bar{Y}}}{\frac{\sigma_x}{\bar{X}}}$.

Singh-Dao (2003) developed a estimator assuming that the existence of information on ρ. It belongs to the subclass determined by $\theta = (0, 1, \rho)$, and is characterized by

$$\bar{y}_{ST} = \frac{\bar{y}}{\bar{x} + \rho} (\overline{X} + \rho)$$

Its MSE is

$$M(\bar{y}_{ST}) = \left(\bar{y}_{razon} \middle| w = \frac{\overline{X}}{\overline{X} + \rho}, \quad \gamma = 2\rho C_y / C_x \right) = \frac{\sigma_y^2 + R^2 \sigma_x^2 \left(\frac{\bar{X}}{\bar{X} + \rho} \right)^2 - 2 \frac{\bar{Y} \rho \sigma_y \sigma_x}{\bar{X} + \rho}}{n}$$

We prefer $\bar{y}_n$ to $\bar{y}_{ST}$ when $\rho < R\sigma_x(w + 1)/\sigma_y$.

Kadilar-Cingi {Kadilar-Cingi 2004 & 2005} analyzed different families of estimators belonging to F identifying them by $\bar{y}(\theta_t)$, where

-

$$\theta_1 = (\alpha_2, B_1, \lambda_1)$$

-

$$\theta_2 = (\alpha_2, B_1, \lambda_3)$$

-

$$\theta_3 = (\alpha_2, B_1, \lambda_4)$$

-

$$\theta_4 = (\alpha_2, B_2, \lambda_1)$$

•

$$\theta_5 = (\alpha_2, B_3, \lambda_3)$$

•

$$\theta_6 = (\alpha_2, B_1, \lambda_2)$$

•

$$\theta_7 = (\alpha_2, B_3 \lambda_2)$$

•

$$\theta_8 = (\alpha_2, B_4, \lambda_4)$$

•

$$\theta_9 = (\alpha_2, B_2, \lambda_2)$$

•

$$\theta_{10} = (\alpha_2, B_4, \lambda_3)$$

Their explícit forms are

$$\bar{y}(\theta_1) = \frac{\bar{y} + b(\bar{X} - \bar{x})}{\bar{x}} \bar{X}, \qquad \bar{y}(\theta_2) = \frac{\bar{y} + b(\bar{X} - \bar{x})}{\bar{x} + B_2(x)} (\bar{X} + B_2(x))$$

$$\bar{y}(\theta_3) = \frac{\bar{y} + b(\bar{X} - \bar{x})}{\bar{x} + C_x} (\bar{X} + C_x), \qquad \bar{y}(\theta_4) = \frac{\bar{y} + b(\bar{X} - \bar{x})}{\bar{x} B_2(x) + C_x} (\bar{X} B_2(x) + C_x)$$

$$\bar{y}(\theta_5) = \frac{\bar{y} + b(\bar{X} - \bar{x})}{\bar{x} C_x + B_2(x)} (\bar{X} C_x + B_2(x)), \qquad \bar{y}(\theta_6) = \frac{\bar{y} + b(\bar{X} - \bar{x})}{\bar{x} + \rho} (\bar{X} + \rho)$$

$$\bar{y}(\theta_7) = \frac{\bar{y} + b(\bar{X} - \bar{x})}{\bar{x} C_x + \rho} (\bar{X} C_x + \rho), \qquad \bar{y}(\theta_8) = \frac{\bar{y} + b(\bar{X} - \bar{x})}{\bar{x} \rho + C_x} (\bar{X} \rho + C_x)$$

$$\bar{y}(\theta_9) = \frac{\bar{y} + b(\bar{X} - \bar{x})}{\bar{x} B_2(x) + \rho} (\bar{X} B_2(x) + \rho), \qquad \bar{y}(\theta_{10}) = \frac{\bar{y} + b(\bar{X} - \bar{x})}{\bar{x} \rho + B_2(x)} (\bar{X} \rho + B_2(x))$$

Their errors are typified by the expression:

$$M(\bar{y}(\theta_t)) = \frac{R^2(\theta_t)\sigma_x^2 + \sigma_y^2(1 - \rho^2)}{n}, \qquad t = 1, \ldots, 10$$

The ratios, indexed by θ_t are defined as:

$$R(\theta_1) = R = \frac{\bar{Y}}{\bar{X}}, \qquad R(\theta_2) = \frac{\bar{Y}}{\bar{X} + B_2(x)}, \qquad R(\theta_3) = \frac{\bar{Y}}{\bar{X} + C_x}, \qquad R(\theta_4) = \frac{\bar{Y}B_2(x)}{\bar{X}B_2(x) + C_x}$$

$$R(\theta_5) = \frac{\bar{Y}C_x}{\bar{X}C_x + B_2(x)}, \qquad R(\theta_6) = \frac{\bar{Y}}{\bar{X} + \rho}, \qquad R(\theta_7) = \frac{\bar{Y}C_x}{\bar{X}C_x + \rho}, \qquad R(\theta_8) = \frac{\bar{Y}\rho}{\bar{X}\rho + C_x},$$

$$R(\theta_9) = \frac{\bar{Y}B_2(x)}{\bar{X}B_2(x) + \rho}, \qquad R(\theta_{10}) = \frac{\bar{Y}B_2(x)}{\bar{X}B_2(x) + \rho},$$

$\bar{y}_n$ is preferred whenever $\rho > \frac{\sigma_x^2 \left(R^2 w^2 - R(\theta_t) \right)}{\sigma_y \left(\sigma_y + 2\sigma_x \right)}$.

Bouza and Al-Omari (2011a) derived RSS versions of these estimators. The RSS- Singh-Deo (2003) estimator developed is

$$\bar{y}_{ST-rss} = \frac{\bar{y}_{rss}}{\bar{x} + \rho} (\bar{X} + \rho)$$

Its MSE is expressed by

$$M(\bar{y}_{ST-rss}) = \frac{\sigma_y^2 - \sum_{i=1}^{m} \frac{\Delta_{Y(i)}^2}{m} + R^2 \left(\sigma_x^2 - \sum_{i=1}^{m} \frac{\Delta_{Y(i)}^2}{m} \right) \left(\frac{\bar{X}}{\bar{X}+\rho} \right)^2 - 2\xi}{n}$$

where

$$\xi = \frac{\bar{Y}\rho \left(\sigma_y^2 - \sum_{i=1}^{m} \frac{\Delta_{Y(i)}^2}{m} \right)^{1/2} \left(\sigma_x^2 - \sum_{i=1}^{m} \frac{\Delta_{Y(i)}^2}{m} \right)^{1/2}}{\bar{X} + \rho}$$

The comparisons of this estimator and the srswr's one fixes to prefer $\bar{y}_{ST-rss}$ if

$$\delta_{ST} = M(\bar{y}_{ST}) - M(\bar{y}_{ST-rss}) > 0 \Rightarrow \sum_{i=1}^{m} \frac{\Delta_{Y(i)}^2}{m} + 2 \frac{\bar{Y}\rho\sigma_y \left(1 - \sum_{i=1}^{m} \frac{\Delta_{Y(i)}^2}{m\sigma_y^2} \right)^{1/.2} \sigma_x}{\bar{X} + \rho} > 0$$

In terms of the correlation is expressed as

$$\rho > -\frac{\bar{X} \sum_{i=1}^{m} \frac{\Delta_{Y(i)}^2}{m}}{\sum_{i=1}^{m} \frac{\Delta_{Y(i)}^2}{m} + 2\bar{Y}\sigma_y \left(1 - \sum_{i=1}^{m} \frac{\Delta_{Y(i)}^2}{m\sigma_y^2} \right)^{1/.2} \sigma}$$

which is generally valid.

A similar study of Kadilar-Cingi (2008) type estimators under RSS permitted to propose the estimators

$$\bar{y}(\theta_{1-\text{rss}}) = \frac{\bar{y}_{\text{rss}} + b(\bar{X} - \bar{x}_{\text{rss}})}{\bar{x}_{\text{rss}}}\mu_X, \quad \bar{y}(\theta_{2-\text{rss}}) = \frac{\bar{y}_{\text{rss}} + b(\bar{X} - \bar{x}_{\text{rss}})}{\bar{x}_{\text{rss}} + B_2(x)}(\mu_X + B_2(x))$$

$$\bar{y}(\theta_{3-\text{rss}}) = \frac{\bar{y}_{\text{rss}} + b(\mu_X - \bar{x}_{\text{rss}})}{\bar{x}_{\text{rss}} + C_{x_{\text{rss}}}}(\mu_X + C_{x_{\text{rss}}}), \quad \bar{y}(\theta_{4-\text{rss}}) = \frac{\bar{y}_{\text{rss}} + b(\mu_X - \bar{x}_{\text{rss}})}{\bar{x}_{\text{rss}}B_2(x) + C_{x_{\text{rss}}}}(\mu_X B_2(x) + C_{x_{\text{rss}}})$$

$$\bar{y}(\theta_{5-\text{rss}}) = \frac{\bar{y}_{\text{rss}} + b(\mu_X - \bar{x}_{\text{rss}})}{\bar{x}C_x + B_2(x)}(\mu_X C_x + B_2(x)), \quad \bar{y}(\theta_{6-\text{rss}}) = \frac{\bar{y}_{\text{rss}} + b(\mu_X - \bar{x}_{\text{rss}})}{\bar{x}_{\text{rss}} + \rho}(\bar{X} + \rho)$$

$$\bar{y}(\theta_{7-\text{rss}}) = \frac{\bar{y}_{\text{rss}} + b(\mu_X - \bar{x}_{\text{rss}})}{\bar{x}_{\text{rss}}C_x + \rho}(\bar{X}C_x + \rho), \quad \bar{y}(\theta_{8-\text{rss}}) = \frac{\bar{y}_{\text{rss}} + b(\mu_X - \bar{x}_{\text{rss}})}{\bar{x}\rho + C_x}(\mu_X \rho + C_x)$$

$$\bar{y}(\theta_{9-\text{rss}}) = \frac{\bar{y}_{\text{rss}} + b(\mu_X - \bar{x}_{\text{rss}})}{\bar{x}_{\text{rss}}B_2(x) + \rho}(\mu_X B_2(x) + \rho), \quad \bar{y}(\theta_{10-\text{rss}}) = \frac{\bar{y}_{\text{rss}} + b(\mu_X - \bar{x}_{\text{rss}})}{\bar{x}_{\text{rss}}\rho + B_2(x)}(\mu_X \rho + B_2(x))$$

The MSE of these RSS estimators of μ_Y has the structure:

$$M(\bar{y}(\theta_{t-\text{rss}})) = \frac{R^2(\theta_{t-\text{rss}})\left[\sigma_x^2 - \sum_{i=1}^{m}\frac{\Delta_{Y(i)}^2}{m}\right] + \left[\sigma_y^2 - \sum_{i=1}^{m}\frac{\Delta_{Y(i)}^2}{m}\right](1 - \rho^2)]}{n}, \quad t = 1, \ldots, 10$$

We prefer them to the srs counterparts whenever
$$M(\bar{y}(\theta_t)) - M(\bar{y}(\theta_{t-\text{rss}})) > 0$$

Say if

$$\delta_t = \frac{R^2(\theta_t)\sum_{i=1}^{m}\frac{\Delta_{X(i)}^2}{m}}{n} + \frac{\sum_{i=1}^{m}\frac{\Delta_{Y(i)}^2}{m}(1 - \rho^2)}{n} > 0, \quad t = 1, .., 10$$

This relationship always holds.

2.4.2 The Difference of Means

Bouza-Prabhu Ajgaonkar (1993) studied the estimation of a difference within the frame proposed by Pi-Ehr (1971). Once a SRSWR is selected from U the difference between the means $D = \mu_Y - \mu_X$ is estimated by

$$D_{srs} = \bar{y} - \bar{x} = \frac{\sum_{i=1}^{n} d_i}{n}, d_i = y_i - x_i$$

Its error is

$$V(D_{srs}) = \frac{\sigma_Y^2 + \sigma_X^2 - 2\rho\sigma_Y\sigma_X}{n}, \rho = \frac{\sigma_{YX}}{\sigma_Y\sigma_X}$$

Bouza (2002b) derived the RSS counterpart. An unbiased estimator of D, when RSS is used is ranking the differences $d_{(i:i)}$.

Using the results derived above, it is easily obtained that when we use RSS and two variables are measured. Ranking the differences an unbiased estimator of D, is

$$D_{rss} = \frac{\sum_{t=1}^{r} \sum_{i=1}^{m} d_{(i:m)t}}{rm}$$

with

$$V(d_{rss}) = \frac{\sigma_d^2}{rm} - \frac{\sum_{i=1}^{m} \Delta_{d(i:m)}^2}{rm^2} = \frac{\sigma_d^2}{n} - \frac{\Delta_d^2}{nm}$$

as variance.

The positiveness of Δ_d^2 grants that the RSS design provides more accurate results than its *srs* counterpart.

References

Abu-dayyeh, W., & Muttlak, H. A. (1996). Usign ranked set samplign for hypothesis test on the scale parameter of the exponential and uniform distributions. *Pakistan Journal of Statistics, 12*, 131–138.

Adatia, A. (2000). Estimation of parameters of the half-logistic distribution using generalized ranked set sampling. *Computational Statistics and Data Analysis, 33*, 1–13.

Al-nasser, D. A. (2007). L-ranked set sampling: a generalization procedure for robust visual sampling. *Communications in Statistics: Simulation and Computation, 6*, 33–43.

Al-omari, A. I, Jaber, k., & Al-omari, A. (2008). Modified ratio-type estimators of the mean using extreme ranked set sampling. *Journal of Mathematics and Statistics, 4*, 150–155.

Al-omari, A. J., Jemain, A. A., & Ibrahim, K. (2009). New ratio estimators of the mean using simple random sampling and ranked set sampling methods. *Revista Investigación Operacional, 30*(2), 97–108.

Al-saleh, M. F. & Al-shrafat, k. (2001). Estimation of average milk ield using randed set sampling. *Environmetrics, 12*, 395-399.I.

Al-Saleh, M.F., & Al-Kadiri, M., (2000). Double ranked set sampling. Statistics and Probability Letters 48: 205–212.

Arnold, B. C., Balakrishnan, N., & Nagaraya, H. N. (1992). *A first course in order statistics.* NewYork: Wiley.

Arnold, B. C., Castillo, E., & Sarabia, J. M. (2009). On multivariate order statistics. Application to ranked set sampling. *Computational Statistics & Data Analysis, 53*, 4555–4569.

Bai, Z. D., & Chen, Z. (2003). On the theory of ranked set sampling *and* its ramifications. *Journal of Statistical Planning and Inference, 109*, 81–99.

Barabesi, I., & El-shamawi, A. (2001). The efficiency of ranked set sampling for parameter estimation. *Statistics and Probability Letters, 53*, 189–199.

Bhoj, D. S. (1997). Estimation of parameters of the extreme value distribution using ranked set sampling. *Communication Statistics Theory and Methods, 26*, 653–667.

Bouza, C. N. (2001a). Model assisted ranked survey sampling. *Biometrical Journal, 43*, 249–259.

Bouza, C. N. (2001b). Ranked set sampling for estimating the differences of means. *Investigación operacional, 22*, 154–162.

Bouza, C. N. (2002b). Ranked set sampling the non-response stratum for estimating the difference of means. *Biometrical Journal, 44*, 903–915.

Bouza, H., Carlos, N., & Al-omari, A. I. (2011a). Ranked set estimation with imputation of the missing observations: the median estimator. *Revista investigación Operacional, 32*, 30–37.

Chen, Z. (1999). Density estimation using ranked set sampling data. *Environment Ecological Statistics, 6*, 135–146.

Chen, Z., & Bai, Z. (2001a). The optimal ranked set sampling for inferences on population quantiles. *Statistica Sinica, 11*, 23–37.

Chen, Z., & Bai, Z. (2001b). Ranked set sampling with regression type estimator. *Journal of Statistical Planning and Inference, 84*, 181–192.

Chen, H., Stasny, E. A., & Wolfe, D. A. (2000). Improved procedures for estimation of disease prevalence using ranked set sampling. *Biometrical Journal, 49*, 530–538.

Chen, Z., Bai, Z., & Sinha, B. K. (2004). *Ranked set sampling : theory and applications. Lectures notes in statistics*. New York: Springer, 176.

Cingi, H., & Kadilar, C. (2005). A new ratio estimator in stratified random sampling. *Communications in Statistics Theory and Methods, 34*, 597–602.

Cobby, J. M., Ridout, M. S., Bassett, P. J., & Large, R. V. (1985). An investigation into the use of ranked set sampling on grass and grass-clover swards. *Grass & Forage Science, 40*, 257–263.

David, H. A., & Levine, D. N. (1972). Ranked set sampling in the presence of judgement error. *Biometrics, 28, 553*–555.

Dell, T. R., & Clutter, J. L. (1972). Ranked set sampling theory with order statistics background. *Biometrics, 28*, 545–555.

Demir, S., & Singh, H. (2000). An application of the regression estimates to ranked set sampling. *Hacettepe Bulletin of Natural Sciences and Engineering Series B, 29*, 93–101.

Gilbert, R. O. (1995). Ranked set sampling. Dqo statistics bulletin: statistical methods for data quality objective process, pnl-sa-26377, The pacific northwest laboratory.

Hall, L. K., & Dell, T. R. (1966). Trials of ranked set sampling for forage yields. *Forest Science. 121,* 22–26.

Hankin, D. G., & Reeves, G. H. (1988). Estimating total fish abundance and total habitat area in small streams based on visual estimation methods. *Canadian Journal of Fisheries and Aquatic Sciences, 45*, 834–844.

Hedayat, A. S., & Sinha, B. K. (1992). *Design and inference in finite population sampling*. New York: Wiley.

Johnson, G. D., Patil, G. P., & Sinha, A. K. (1993). Ranked set sampling for vegetation research. *Abstract Botanical, 17*, 87–102.

Kadilar, C., & Cingi, H. (2004). Ratio estimators in simple random sampling. *Applied Mathematics and Computatio,151*, 893-902.

Kadilar, C., & Cingi, H. (2008). Estimators for the population mean in the case of missing data. *Communication in Statistics Theory and Methods, 37*, 2226–2236.

Kaur, A., Patil, G. P., Shiek, J., & Taillie, C. (1996). Environmental sampling with a concomitant variable: a comparison between ranked set sampling and stratified random sampling. *Journal of Applied Statistical Science, 23*, 231–255.

Kaur, A., Patil, G.P., & Taillie, C. (1997). Unequal allocation models for ranked set sampling with skew distributions. Biometrics 53: 123–130.

Lehmann, E. L. (1966). Some concepts of dependence. *The Annals of Mathematical Statistics, 37*, 1137–1153.

Martin, W. L., Sharik, T. L., Oderwald, R. G., & Smith, D. W. (1980*). Evaluation of ranked set sampling for estimating shrub phytomass in appalachian oak forests, publication number fws-4-80*. Blacksburg, Virginia: School of Forestry and Wildlife Resources, Virginia Polytechnic Institute and State University.

Mc intyre, G. A. (1952). A method of unbiased selective sampling using ranked sets. *Journal of Agricultural Research, 3*, 385–390.

Mcintyre, G. A. (1978). *Statistical aspects of vegetation sampling. Measurement of grassland vegetation and animal production* (pp. 8–21). Hurley, Berkshire, UK: Commonwealth Bureau of Pastures and Field Crops.

Ahmad, M., Muhammad, H., & Muttlak, H. A., and contributors (2010). *Ranked set sampling.* newcastle upon tyne: cambridge scholars publishing.

Muttlak, H. A. (1995). Median ranked set sampling. *Journal of Applied Statistical Science., 6,* 91–98.

Muttlak, H. A. (1998). Median ranked set sampling with size biased probability selection. *Biometrical Journal, 40,* 455–465.

Muttlak, H. A. (2003). Investigating the use of quartile ranked set samples for estimating the population mean. *Journal of Applied Mathematics and Computation, 146,* 437.

Muttlak, H. A., & Mcdonald, I. D. (1992). Ranked set sampling and the line intercept method: a more efficient procedure. *Biometrical Journal, 34*(3), 329–346.

Nussbaum, B. D., & Sinha, B. K. (1997). Cost effective gasoline sampling using ranked set sampling. *ASA Proceedings of the Section on Statistics and the Environment* (pp. 83–87).

Patil, G. P., Sinha, A. K., & Taillie, C. (1995). Finite corrections for ranked set sampling. *Annals of the Institute of Mathematical Statistics, Tokyo, 47,* 621–636.

Patil, G. P., Sinha, A. K., & Taillie, C. (1997a). Median ranked set sampling. *Journal of Applied Statistical Science, 6,* 245–255.

Patil, G. P., Sinha, A. K., & Taillie, C. (1997b). Ranked set sampling coherent ranking and size biased permutation. *Journal of Statistical Planning and Inference, 63,* 311–324.

Pi-Ehr, L. (1971). Estimation procedures for the difference of means with missing observations. *Journal of the American Statistical Association, 41,* 517–529.

Samawi, H. M., & Muttlak H. A. (1996). Estimation of a ratio using ranked set sampling. *Biometrical Journal, 36,* 753–764.

Samawi, H., Abu-dayyeh, W., & Ahmed, S. (1996a). Extreme ranked set sampling. *Biometrical Journal, 30,* 577–586.

Samawi, H. M., Ahmed, M. S. & Abu Dayyeh, W. A. (1996). Estimating the population mean using extreme ranked set sampling. *Biomtrical Journal, 38,* 577–586.

Singh, S., & Deo, B. (2003). Imputation by power transformation. *Statistical Papers, 44,* 555–579.

Sinha, B. K., Sinha, A. K., & Purkayasthra, S. (1996). On some aspects of ranked set sampling for estimation of normal and exponential parameters. *Statistics and Decisions, 14,* 223–240.

Stokes, S. L. (1977a). Ranked set sampling with concomitant variable. *Communication in Statistics: Theory and Methods, 6,* 1207–1211.

Stokes, S. L. (1977b). Ranked set sampling with concomitant variable. *Communication in Statistics: Theory and Methods, 6,* 1207–1211.

Stokes, S. L. (1980). Estimation of the variance using judgment ordered ranked set samples. *Biometrics, 36,* 35–42.

Takahasi, K., & Fututsuya, M. (1998). Dependence between order statistics in samples from finite population and its applications to ranked set sampling. *Annals Internal Mathematics and Statistics, 50,* 49–70.

Takahasi, K., & Wakimoto, K. (1968). On unbiased estimates of population mean based on the sample stratified by means of ordering. *Internship in Mathematics and Statistics, 20,* 1–31.

Yanagawa, T. (2000). K. Wakimoto's contribution to ranked set sampling. *The Tenth Japan-Korea Joint Conference in Statistics,* 179–184.

Yu, P. L. H., & Lam k. (1997). Regression estimator in ranked set sampling. *Biometrics, 53,* 1070–1080.

Chapter 3
The Non-response Problem: Subsampling Among the Non-respondents

Abstract The existence of missing observations in the estimation problems present in random sampling can be considered unimportant. But the risk of misunderstanding is high because the non-responses may be generated by the existence of a very different behavior of a group of units. This is especially important when human populations are sampled. The solution of subsampling among the non-respondents is the most intelligent approach in such cases. The usual simple random sampling models are revisited and their ranked set sample counterpart developed. Generally they are more accurate.

Keywords Non-respondent's strata · Subsampling rules · Expected variance · SRS · RSS · Efficiency

> *See all, conceal much, modify little.*
> Gregorio Magno

3.1 Some Aspects of Non-response

As quoted the usual theory of survey sampling is developed assuming that the finite population $U = \{u_1,...,u_N\}$ is composed of individuals that can be perfectly identified. A sample s of size $n \leq N$ is selected. The variable of interest Y is measured in each selected unit. Real life surveys should deal with the existence of missing observations. Non-responses may be motivated by a refusal of some units to give the true value of Y or by other causes. Refusals to respond are present in the majority of the surveys. There are three solutions to cope with this fact: ignore the non-respondents to subsample the non-respondents or to impute the missing values. To ignore the non-responses is a dangerous decision, to subsample is a conservative and costly solution, see Cochran (1977), Bouza (1981a, b, 2001). Imputation is often used to compensate for item non-response. See for discussions on the theme Singh (2003), Särndal and Lundström (2005) for example.

C. N. Bouza-Herrera, *Handling Missing Data in Ranked Set Sampling*,
SpringerBriefs in Statistics, DOI: 10.1007/978-3-642-39899-5_3,
© The Author(s) 2013

The existence of non-responses does not permit to compute the sample mean

$$\bar{y} = \frac{\sum_{i=1}^{n} y_i}{n}$$

which estimates the population mean μ because we obtain response only from the units in $s_1 = \{i \in s | i$ *gives a response at the first visit*$\}$.

This fact suggests that the population U is divided into two strata: U_1, where are grouped the units giving a response at the first visit, and U_2 which contains the rest of the individuals. This is the so-called 'response strata' model and was first proposed by Hansen-Hurvitz (1946), see Cochran (1977), Singh (2003). They proposed to select a subsample s'_2 of size n'_2 among the n_2 non-respondents grouped in the sample s_2. When subsampling the non-respondents the researcher contacts a subsample of the non-respondents, usually by means of telephone or personal interviews.

Then we obtain information on the non-respondent's strata U_2 through s'_2

3.2 Estimation of the Mean

Non-responses may be motivated by a refusal of some units to give the true value of Y or by other causes. Hansen-Hurvitz in 1946 proposed selecting a sub-sample among the non-respondents, see Cochran (1977), Singh (2003), Särndal and Lundström (2005), Singh-Kumar (2008a). The idea is that we select a sample from the population U without knowing that it is stratified into U_1, stratum of the units to give a response at the first visit, and U_2 the stratum that contains the rest of the units. The mean of the variable of interest is

$$\mu_Y = \frac{\sum_{i=1}^{2} \sum_{j \in U_i} Y_j}{N} = \sum_{i=1}^{2} W_i \frac{\sum_{j \in U_i} Y_j}{N_i} = \sum_{i=1}^{2} W_i \mu_{Y(i)}, W_i = \frac{N_i}{N}, i = 1, 2.$$

It is supposed that the non-responses are due to the fact that the units in U_2 have a behavior different of those in U_1 and that it affects the values of Y in such a way that the strata means are different.

Take s as the initial sample and $s_i \subset U_i$, with size n_i. A sub-sample of size $n'_2 = \theta n_2$ is selected among the non-respondents and a response is obtained from them. This feature depends heavily on the sub-sampling rule. Some sub-sampling rules have been proposed by Hansen-Hurvitz (1946), Srinath (1971) and Bouza (1981b). The rule of Hansen-Hurvitz uses

$$\text{RHH} : \theta = 1/K, K > 1$$

The proposal of Srinath (1971) was to set

$$\text{RS} : \theta = \frac{n_2}{Hn + n_2}, H > 0$$

The rule of Bouza (1981b) is

$$\text{RB} : \theta = \frac{n_2}{n}$$

As this rule is randomized the surveyor does not have to fix an arbitrary value of θ.

The sampling procedure is a particular case of double sampling design described as follows:

Step 1: Select a sample s from U and evaluate Y among the respondents determine

$$\{y_i : i \in s_1 \subseteq U_1 : |s_1| = n_1\}.$$

Step 2: Determine $n_2' = \theta n_2, 0 < \theta < 1; /s_2/ = n_2$ with $s_2 = s \backslash s_1$.

Step 3: Select a sub-sample s''_2 of size n'_2' from s_2 and evaluate Y among the units in $s'_2, \{y_i : i \in s'_2; s'_2 \subset s_2, s_2 \subseteq U_2\}$.

Step 4: Compute $\bar{y}_1 = \frac{\sum_{i=1}^{n_1} y_i}{n_1}, \bar{y}'_2 = \frac{\sum_{i=1}^{n'_2} y_i}{n'_2}.,$ and   the   estimate   of μ is
$\bar{\bar{y}} = \frac{n_1}{n}\bar{y}_1 + \frac{n_2}{n}\bar{y}'_2 = w_1\bar{y}_1 + w_2\bar{y}'_2$

Note that $\bar{y}_1$ is the mean of a SRSWR-sample selected from U_1, the response stratum, then its expected value is the mean of Y in the respondent stratum: $\mu_{Y(1)}$.

We have the conditional expectation of $\bar{y}'_2 = \frac{\sum_{i=1}^{n'_2} y_i}{n'_2}$ is

$$E[\bar{y}'_2|s] = \bar{y}_2$$

as it is the mean of a SRSWR-sample selected from the non-response stratum U_2

$$EE[\bar{y}'_2|s] = \mu_{Y(2)}$$

Taking into account that for $i = 1,2$ $E(n_i) = nW_i$ the unbiasedness of $\bar{\bar{y}}$ is easily derived.

The variance of the estimator can be deduced using the following trick
$\bar{\bar{y}} = (w_1\bar{y}_1 + w_2\bar{y}_2) + w_2(\bar{y}'_2 - \bar{y}_2)$.

The first term is the mean of Y in s, and then its variance is σ^2/n. For the second term we have that

$$V\left(w_2(\bar{y}'_2 - \bar{y}_2)|s\right) = w_2^2 E\left(\bar{y}'_2 - \mu_{Y(2)}) - (\bar{y}_2 - \mu_{Y(2)})|s\right)^2$$

$$= w_2^2\left[E\left(\bar{y}'_2 - \mu_{Y(2)})|s\right)^2 + E\left((\bar{y}_2 - \mu_{Y(2)})|s\right)^2\right.$$

$$\left. - 2E\left(\bar{y}'_2 - \mu_{Y(2)})\left((\bar{y}_2 - \mu_{Y(2)})\right)|s\right)\right]$$

Conditioning to a fixed n_2 we have that the expectation of the third term is $(\bar{y}_2 - \mu_{Y(2)})^2$. Then we have that:

$$V\left(w_2\left(\bar{y}_2' - \bar{y}_2\right)|s\right) = w_2^2\left(\frac{\sigma_{Y(2)}^2}{n_2'} - \frac{\sigma_{Y(2)}^2}{n_2}\right) = w_2^2\sigma_{Y(2)}^2\left(\frac{1-\theta}{\theta n_2}\right)$$

For the different rules we have

$$EV\left(w_2\left(\bar{y}_2' - \bar{y}_2\right)|s\right) = \begin{cases} \text{If } RHH \text{ is used} & \frac{W_2(K-1)\sigma_{Y(2)}^2}{n} \\ \text{If } RS \text{ is used} & \frac{H\sigma_{Y(2)}^2}{n} \\ \text{If } RB \text{ is used} & \frac{W_1\sigma_{Y(2)}^2}{n} \end{cases}$$

We will use in the sequel

$$\varpi = \begin{cases} W_2(K-1) & \text{if } RHH \quad \text{is used} \\ H\,k & \text{if } RS \quad \text{is used} \\ W_1 & \text{if } RB \quad \text{is used} \end{cases}$$

as the factor of $\sigma_{Y(2)}^2$.

This discussion sustains the validity of the following proposition.

Corollary 3.1 *Consider that a sample of size n is selected from a finite population of size stratified into a response stratum U_1 of size N_1 and a non-responses stratum U_2 of size N_2. If a SRSWR is selected among the non-respondents an unbiased estimator of the population mean μ_Y is*

$$\bar{\bar{y}} = w_1\bar{y}_1 + w_2\bar{y}_2, \quad w_i = \frac{n_i}{n}, \quad i = 1, 2, \quad \bar{y}_1 = \frac{\sum_{i=1}^{n_1} y_i}{n_1}, \quad \bar{y}_2' = \frac{\sum_{i=1}^{n_2'} y_i}{n_2'}$$

and its expected variance is

$$EV(\bar{y}) = \frac{\sigma_Y^2}{n} + \frac{\varpi\sigma_{Y(2)}^2}{n}$$

$\square$

3.3 RSS Designs and the Non-responses

3.3.1 Managing with NR

Commonly the sample is selected using SRSWR. A sample s is selected and the units in the sample are visited for obtaining information on Y. The units which can not be interviewed at the first visit are revisited, and the surveyor obtains some information on them. This information allows ranking the non-respondents. This procedure permits to use a smaller sample size, as RSS is more precise than SRSWR, for the same error fixed and accepted for deriving the initial sample size. We will consider the usage of a RSS procedure for sub-sampling s_2. We take a subsample $s'_{2(RSS)}$ from s using RSS. That is, we select n'_2 independent samples of size $n'_2 = \theta n_2$ using SRSWR. The units are ranked accordingly with the variable closely related with the variable of interest Y collected at the first visit.

3.3.2 The Use of RSS for Subsampling s_2

As RSS provides more reliable estimations of the population mean it seems that to use it for subsampling the non-respondent stratum would provide a better alternative than to use again SRSWR.

$$Y_{11}, Y_{12} \ldots, Y_{1n'_2}; Y_{21}, Y_{22} \ldots, Y_{2n'_2}; \ldots; Y_{n'_2 1}, Y_{n'_2 2} \ldots, Y_{n'_2 n'_2}$$

Take the n'_2 independent random samples.

They are ranked and we obtain

$$Y_{(1:1)}, Y_{(2:1)} \ldots, Y_{(n'_2:1)}; Y_{(1:2)}, Y_{(2:2)} \ldots, Y_{(n'_2:2)}; \ldots; Y_{(n'_2:1)}, Y_{(n'_2:2)} \ldots, Y_{(n'_2:n'_2)}$$

where $Y_{(j:t)}$ is the j-th order statistic (os) in the sample of size m of the t-th sample, $j = 1,\ldots,n'_2$, and $t = 1,\ldots,n'_2$. As usual the RSS sample is formed by the n'_2 os in the diagonal. That is the measurements of Y are

$$Y_{(1:1)}, Y_{(2:2)} \ldots, Y_{(n'_2:n'_2)}$$

The estimate of the mean of the non-respondent stratum is made by using the estimator:

$$\bar{y}'_{2(\text{rss})} = \frac{\sum_{j=1}^{n'_2} Y_{(j:j)}}{n'_2}$$

The behavior of this model is characterized in the following proposition.

Proposition 3.2 *Consider that a sample of size n is selected from a finite population of size N stratified into a response stratum U_1 of size N_1 and a non-responses stratum U_2 of size N'_2 If a RSS sample of size n'_2 is selected among the nonrespondents an unbiased estimator of the population mean μ_Y is s*

$$\bar{\bar{y}}_{(\text{rss})} = \frac{n_1}{n}\bar{y}_1 + \frac{n_2}{n}\bar{y}'_{2(\text{rss})} = w_1\bar{y}_1 + w_2\bar{y}'_{2(\text{rss})}$$

and

$$EV(\bar{\bar{y}}_{(rss)}) = \frac{\sigma_Y^2}{n} + \frac{\varpi\sigma_{Y(2)}^2}{n} - E\left(\frac{\sum\limits_{j=1}^{n_2'} \Delta_{Y(j)}^2}{\upsilon}\right)$$

where

$$\upsilon = \begin{cases} \dfrac{n}{W_2 K} & \text{if } RHH \text{ is used} \\[2mm] \dfrac{n^2}{Hn + n^2} & \text{if } RS \text{ is used} \\[2mm] n & \text{if } RB \text{ is used} \end{cases}$$

Proof First note that $E[Y_{(j:j)} | n_2] = \mu_{(j)}, j = 1,\dots,n'_2$. At this randomization stage the parameter of interest is the mean of Y in s_2. The RSS estimator of the non-respondents mean is unbiased:

$$E\left(\bar{y}'_{2(rss)}\right) = E\left(\frac{\sum\limits_{j=1}^{n_2'} E\left(Y_{(j:j)}\right)}{n'_2}\right) = E[\bar{y}_2] = \mu_{Y(2)}$$

We may write $\bar{\bar{y}}_{(rss)} = (w_1\bar{y}_1 + w_2\bar{y}_2) + w_2\left(\bar{y}'_{2(rss)} - \bar{y}_2\right)$.

Its conditional variance is $V(\bar{\bar{y}}_{(rss)} | s) = \frac{\sigma_{Y(2)}^2}{n} + w_2^2 V\left(\bar{y}'_{2(rss)} - \bar{y}_2 | s\right)$. We needed to obtain an explicit expression of the second term in the right-hand side. It is:

$$V\left(w_2\left(\bar{y}'_2 - \bar{y}_2\right) | s\right) = w_2^2 E\left(\left(\bar{y}'_{2(rss)} - \mu_{Y(2)}\right) - (\bar{y}_2 - \mu_{Y(2)}) | s\right)^2$$

$$= w_2^2\left[E\left(\left(\bar{y}'_{2(rss)} - \mu_{Y(2)}\right) | s\right)^2 + E\left((\bar{y}_2 - \mu_{Y(2)}) | s\right)^2\right.$$

$$\left. - 2E\left(\left(\bar{y}'_{2(rss)} - \mu_{Y(2)}\right)(\bar{y}_2 - \mu_{Y(2)}) | s\right)\right]$$

The first term of the equation within brackets is equal to

$$\frac{\sum\limits_{j=1}^{n_2'} \Delta_{Y(j)}^2}{n'_2} = \frac{\sum\limits_{j=1}^{n_2'} (\mu_{Y(j)} - \mu_Y)^2}{n'_2} - E\left(\left(\bar{y}'_{2(rss)} - \mu_{Y(2)}\right)\right) | s^2 = \frac{\sum\limits_{j=1}^{n_2'} \sigma_{Y(j)}^2}{n'_2} = \frac{\sigma_{Y(2)}^2}{n'_2} - \frac{\sum\limits_{j=1}^{n_2'} \Delta_{Y(j)}^2}{n'_2}$$

where
Then

$$E\Big(E[(\bar{y}'_{2(\mathrm{rss})} - \mu_{Y(2)})]\big((\bar{y}_2 - \mu_{Y(2)})\big)|s\Big) = E\Big(\big((\bar{y}_2 - \mu_{Y(2)})\big)^2|s\Big) = \frac{\sigma^2_{Y(2)}}{n_2}$$

The second term of $V\big(w_2(\bar{y}'_2 - \bar{y}_2)|s\big)$ is related to the use of SRSWR for selecting s_2 and it is equal to

$$E\Big((\bar{y}_2 - \mu_{Y(2)})|s\Big)^2 = \frac{\sigma^2_{Y(2)}}{n_2}$$

Hence the counterpart of $V\big(w_2(\bar{y}'_2 - \bar{y}_2)|s\big)$ is

$$V\Big(w_2\big(\bar{y}'_{2(\mathrm{rss})} - \bar{y}_2\big)|s\Big) = w_2^2\left(\frac{\sigma^2_{Y(2)(\mathrm{rss})}}{n'_2} - \frac{\sigma^2_{Y(2)}}{n_2}\right) = w_2^2\left(\frac{\sigma^2_{Y(2)}}{n'_2} - \frac{\sigma^2_{Y(2)}}{n_2} - \frac{\displaystyle\sum_{j=1}^{n'_2}\Delta^2_{Y(j)}}{n'_2}\right)$$

$$(3.4)$$

Substituting $n'_2 = \theta n_2$ we derived that the two first terms are equal to $V\big(w_2(\bar{y}'_2 - \bar{y}_2)|s\big)$ and we obtain the stated results. □

The proposed model is more accurate that the use of SRSWR for subsampling the non-respondents because

$$E\left(\frac{\displaystyle\sum_{j=1}^{n'_2}\Delta^2_{Y(j)}}{v}\right) \geq 0.$$

Computing the involved expectation is rather complicated as the n'_2 is a random variable.

It is clear that if the procedure is applied for r RSS samples of size m'_2, $n'_2 = rm'_2$, the following corollary is easily derived.

Corollary 3.3 *Under the conditions of the previous proposition when $n'_2 = \theta rm_2$, $r > 1$, substituting*

$$\bar{y}'_{2(\mathrm{rss})} = \frac{\displaystyle\sum_{t=1}^{r}\sum_{j=1}^{m'_2} Y_{(j:j)t}}{rm'_2}$$

in

$$\bar{\bar{y}}_{(\text{rss})} = \frac{n_1}{n}\bar{y}_1 + \frac{n_2}{n}\bar{y}'_{2(\text{rss})} = w_1\bar{y}_1 + w_2\bar{y}'_{2(\text{rss})}$$

is

$$EV(\bar{\bar{y}}_{(\text{rss})}) = \frac{\sigma^2}{n} + \frac{\varpi\sigma_2^2}{n} - E\left(\frac{\sum_{j=1}^{n'_2}\Delta^2_{Y_{(j)}}}{vr}\right),$$

3.3.3 The Use of the Extreme RSS for Subsampling s_2

Extreme RSS has a practical sound basis because the surveyor can be interested only in the extreme behavior of Y among the non-respondents. In addition, it is easier to identify them in the first visit as to rank all the units may be subject to large errors. Some further considerations can be obtained in Samawi-Abu-Dayyeh-Ahmed (1996):

Considering that n'_2 is even when we evaluate only the extremes in the subsample among the non-respondents

$$Y_{2(j:e)} = \frac{Y_{2(j:1)} + Y_{2(j:n'_2)}}{2}$$

An estimator of the mean in U_2 is:

$$\bar{y}'_{2(\text{rss})} = \frac{\sum_{j=1}^{n'_2}Y_{2(j:e)}}{n'_2} = \frac{Y_{2(1)} + Y_{2(n'_2)}}{2}$$

Hence we have that

$$E(\bar{y}'_{2(\text{erss})}) = \frac{\mu_{2(1)} + \mu_{2(n'_2)}}{2} = \mu_{2(e)}$$

For n odd we introduce the variable

$$Y_{2(j:e)} = \begin{cases} \frac{Y_{2(j:1)} + Y_{2(j:n'_2)}}{2} & \text{if} \quad j = n'_2 \\ Y_{2(j:1)} & \text{if} \quad j < n'_2 \quad j \quad \text{odd} \\ Y_{2(j:n'_2)} & \text{if} \quad j < n'_2 \quad j \quad \text{even} \end{cases}$$

and

$$
E(Y_{2(j:e)}) = \begin{cases} \dfrac{\mu_{2(1)}+\mu_{2(n'_2)}}{2} & \text{if} \quad j=n'_2 \\ \mu_{2(1)} & \text{if} \quad j<n'_2 \quad j \quad \text{odd} \\ \mu_{2(n'_2)} & \text{if} \quad j<n'_2 \quad j \quad \text{even} \end{cases}
$$

Hence, it is possible using the estimator

$$
\bar{y}'_{2(\text{erss})} = \frac{\sum\limits_{j=1}^{n'_2} Y_{2(j:e)}}{n'_2}
$$

and it has the same expectation as in the even case but a different variance. Previously, in Chap. 2 we have derived that this estimator is biased. If the distribution is symmetric with respect to $\mu_{Y(2)}$, its bias

$$
B(\bar{y}'_{2(\text{erss})}) = \frac{\left(\mu_{Y(2)(1)} - \mu_{Y(2)}\right) + \left(\mu_{Y(2)(n'_2)} - \mu_{Y(2)}\right)}{2}
$$

is equal to zero. Then the symmetry of the distribution plays a role in the magnitude of the bias. The variance of the involved os's are $\sigma^2_{Y(2)(1)}$ and $\sigma^2_{Y(2)(n'_2)}$. Then

$$
V\left(\bar{y}'_{2(\text{erss})}\right) = \begin{cases} \dfrac{\sigma^2_{Y(2)(1)}+\sigma^2_{Y(2)(n'_2)}}{2n'_2} = \dfrac{\sigma^2_{Y(2)}}{n'_2} - \dfrac{\Delta^2_{(e)}}{2n'_2} & \text{if} \quad n'_2 \quad \text{even} \\[3ex] \dfrac{(2n'_2-1)\left(\sigma^2_{Y(2)(1)}+\sigma^2_{Y(2)(n'_2)}\right)+2\sigma_{(1,n)}}{4n'^2_2} = \dfrac{(2n'_2-1)(\sigma^2_{Y(2)}-\Delta^2_{(e)})}{4n'^2_2} + \dfrac{\sigma_{(1,n)}}{n'^2_2} & \\[2ex] & \text{if} \quad n'_2 \quad \text{odd} \end{cases}
$$

$$
\Delta^2_{(e)} = \Delta^2_{Y(2)(1)} + \Delta^2_{Y(2)\left(n'_2\right)}, \quad 2\sigma_{(1,n)} = Cov\left(Y_{2\left(1:n'_2\right)}, Y_{2\left(n'_2:n'_2\right)}\right)
$$

with $\Delta_{Y(2)(1)} = \mu_{Y(2)(1)} - \mu_{Y(2)}$ and $\Delta_{Y(2)\left(n'_2\right)} = \mu_{Y(2)(n_2)} - \mu_{Y(2)}$. We may use the estimator

$$
\bar{\bar{y}}_{(\text{erss})} = w_1\bar{y}_1 + w_2\bar{y}'_{2(\text{erss})} = \bar{y} + w_2\left(\bar{y}'_{2(\text{erss})} - \bar{y}_2\right)
$$

Its bias is $W_2B(ERSS)$. The general expression of the variance is

$$
V(\bar{\bar{y}}_{(\text{erss})}) = V(\bar{y}_1) + w^2_2 E(\bar{y}'_{2(\text{erss})} - \bar{y}_2|s)^2
$$

Considering the relationships used for deriving the expectation of the conditional variance we have that in the even case

$$w_2^2\left(\frac{\sigma_{Y(2)}^2}{n_2'} - \frac{\Delta_{(e)}^2}{2n_2'}\right) = \frac{n_2}{n^2}\left(\frac{\sigma_{Y(2)}^2}{\theta} - \frac{\Delta_{(e)}^2}{2\theta}\right)$$

Hence

$$E(V(\bar{\bar{y}}_{(erss)})) = \frac{\sigma^2}{n} + \frac{W_2}{n}\left(\frac{\sigma_{Y(2)}^2}{\theta} - \frac{\Delta_{(e)}^2}{2\theta}\right) \quad \text{if} \quad n_2' \quad \text{is} \quad \text{even}$$

For the odd case we have

$$w_2^2\left(\frac{(2n_2'-1)(\sigma_{Y(2)}^2 - \Delta_{(e)}^2) + 4\sigma_{(1,n)}}{4n_2'^2}\right) = \frac{1}{n^2}\left(\frac{(2n_2\theta - 1)(\sigma_{Y(2)}^2 - \Delta_{(e)}^2) + 4\sigma_{(1,n)}}{4\theta^2}\right)$$

Therefore if RHH: $\theta = 1/K$, $K > 1$ is used

$$E(V(\bar{\bar{y}}_{(erss)})) = \frac{\sigma^2}{n} + \frac{K(2W_2 - K)(\sigma_{Y(2)}^2 - \Delta_{(e)}^2) + 4K^2\sigma_{(1,n)}}{4n^2}$$

When it is considered RS : $\theta = \frac{n_2}{Hn+n_2}$, $H > 0$

$$w_2^2\left(\frac{(2n_2'-1)(\sigma_{Y(2)}^2 - \Delta_{(e)}^2) + 4\sigma_{(1,n)}}{4n_2'^2}\right) = \frac{1}{n^2}\left(\frac{(\frac{2n_2^2}{Hn+n_2} - 1)(\sigma_{Y(2)}^2 - \Delta_{(e)}^2) + 4\sigma_{(1,n)}}{\left(\frac{2n_2}{Hn+n_2}\right)^2}\right)$$

This results permit to establish the following proposition.

Proposition 3.4 *Consider the use of extreme RSS and*

$$Y_{2(j:e)} = \begin{cases} \frac{Y_{2(j:1)} + Y_{2(j:n_2')}}{2} & \text{if} \quad j = n_2' \quad \text{and} \quad \text{odd} \quad \text{or} \quad n_2' \quad \text{is} \quad \text{even} \\ Y_{2(j:1)} & \text{if} \quad n_2' \quad \text{and} \quad j < n_2' \quad \text{are} \quad \text{odd} \\ Y_{2(j:n_2')} & \text{if} \quad n_2' \quad \text{is} \quad \text{odd} \quad \text{and} \quad j < n_2' \quad \text{is} \quad \text{even} \end{cases}$$

$$\bar{\bar{y}}_{(erss)} = w_1\bar{y}_1 + w_2\bar{y}_{2(erss)}', \quad \bar{y}_{2(erss)}' = \frac{\sum_{j=1}^{n_2'} Y_{2(j:e)}}{n_2'}, n_2' = \theta n_2$$

has bias

$$B(\bar{y}_{2(erss)}') = \frac{\left(\mu_{Y(2)(1)} - \mu_{Y(2)}\right) + \left(\mu_{Y(2)(n_2')} - \mu_{Y(2)}\right)}{2}$$

and expected variance

$$E(V(\bar{\bar{y}}_{(erss)})) = \begin{cases} \frac{\sigma^2}{n} + \frac{W_2}{n}\left(\frac{\sigma^2_{Y(2)}}{\theta} - \frac{\Delta^2_{(e)}}{2\theta}\right) & \text{if } n_2' \text{ is even} \\ \frac{\sigma^2}{n} + \frac{(2W_2\theta-1)(\sigma^2_{Y(2)}-\Delta^2_{(e)})+4\sigma_{(1,n)}}{4n^2\theta^2} & \text{if } n_2' \text{ is odd} \end{cases}$$

$\square$

3.3.4 The Use of Median RSS for Subsampling s_2

Muttlak (1996) proposed using Median RSS. Let us define an operational variable

$$Y^*_{2(j:med)} = \begin{cases} Y_{2\left(j:\frac{n_2'+1}{2}\right)} & \text{if } n_2' \text{ odd} \\ Y_{2\left(j:\frac{n_2'}{2}\right)} & \text{if } n_2' \text{ even } \quad j = 1, 2, \ldots, n_2'/2 \\ Y_{2\left(j:\frac{n_2'+2}{2}\right)} & \text{if } n_2' \text{ even } \quad j = \frac{n_2'}{2}+1, \ldots, n_2' \end{cases}$$

$$\bar{y}'_{2(mrss)} = \frac{\sum\limits_{j=1}^{n_2'} Y^*_{2(j:med)}}{n_2'}$$

and

$$E\left(\bar{y}'_{2(mrss)}\right) = \begin{cases} \mu_{\left(\frac{n_2'+1}{2}\right)} & \text{if } n_2' \text{ is odd} \\ \frac{1}{2}\left(\mu_{\left(\frac{n_2'}{2}\right)} + \mu_{\left(\frac{n_2'}{2}+1\right)}\right) & \text{if } n_2' \text{ is even} \end{cases}$$

An estimator of the non-responses based on the subsample is
The variances of the random variables which are

$$V(Y_{2(j:m)}) = \begin{cases} \sigma^2_{2\left(\frac{n_2'+1}{2}\right)} & \text{if } n_2' \text{ is odd} \\ \sigma^2_{2\left(\frac{n_2'}{2}\right)} & \text{if } n_2' \text{ is even } \quad \text{and } j = 1, \ldots, \frac{n_2'}{2} \\ \sigma^2_{2\left(\frac{n_2'+2}{2}\right)} & \text{if } n_2' \text{ is even } \quad \text{and } j = \frac{n_2'}{2}+1, \ldots, n_2' \end{cases}$$

Consider the odd case

$$V(\bar{y}'_{2(\mathrm{mrss})}) = \frac{\sum_{j=1}^{n'_2} V(Y_{2(j:m)})}{n'^2_2} = \frac{\sigma^2_{2\left(\frac{n'_2+1}{2}\right)}}{n'_2} = \frac{\sigma^2_2}{n'_2} - \frac{\Delta^2_{2\left(\frac{n'_2+1}{2}\right)}}{n'_2}$$

In the even case

$$V(\bar{y}'_{2(\mathrm{mrss})}) = \frac{\sum_{j=1}^{n'_2} V(Y_{2(j:m)})}{n'^2_2} = \frac{\sigma^2_{2\left(\frac{n'_2}{2}\right)} + \sigma^2_{2\left(\frac{n'_2+2}{2}\right)}}{2n'_2} = \frac{\sigma^2_2}{n'_2} - \frac{\Delta^2_{2\left(\frac{n'_2}{2}\right)} + \Delta^2_{2\left(\frac{n'_2+2}{2}\right)}}{2n'_2}$$

$$= \frac{\sigma^2_2}{n'_2} - \frac{\Delta^2_{2(m)}}{2n'_2}$$

The estimators is biased because

$$E(\bar{y}'_{2(\mathrm{mrss})}) = \begin{cases} \mu_{2\left(\frac{n'_2+1}{2}\right)} & \text{if } n'_2 \text{ is odd} \\[2ex] \dfrac{\mu_{2\left(\frac{n'_2}{2}\right)} + \mu_{2\left(\frac{n'_2+2}{2}\right)}}{2} & \text{if } n'_2 \text{ is even} \end{cases}$$

When we deal with distributions symmetric with respect to μ_2, we may expect that it will be close to the median. A good example is the normal distribution where the median and mean coincides. In general the bias is:

$$(B(\mathrm{mrss})) = \begin{cases} \mu_{2\left(\frac{n'_2+1}{2}\right)} & \text{if } n'_2 \text{ is odd} \\[2ex] \dfrac{\left(\mu_{2\left(\frac{n'_2}{2}\right)} - \mu_2\right) + \left(\mu_{2\left(\frac{n'_2+2}{2}\right)} - \mu_2\right)}{2} & \text{if } n'_2 \text{ is even} \end{cases}$$

The estimator of the overall mean is derived from the general expression. It is

$$\bar{\bar{y}}_{(\mathrm{mrss})} = w_1 \bar{y}_1 + w_2 \bar{y}'_{2(\mathrm{mrss})}$$

It is easily derived that its expected variance for the even case is:

$$EV(\bar{\bar{y}}_{2(\mathrm{mrss})}) = \frac{\sigma^2}{n} + \frac{\varpi \sigma^2_2}{n} - \frac{E\left(\Delta^2_{(m)}\right)}{2\upsilon}$$

Then we have proven the following proposition.

Proposition 3.5 *Select an RSS subsample from s_2' of size n_2' and measure $Y_{2(j:med)}^*$.*
The RSS median estimator of the population mean $\bar{y}_{2(MRSS)}'$ with expected variance

$$EV(\overset{=}{\underset{2(mrss)}{y}}) = \frac{\sigma^2}{n} + \frac{\varpi\sigma_2^2}{n} - \frac{W_2 E\left(\Delta_{(m)}^2\right)}{2\upsilon}$$

and expected error

$$\Delta_{(m)}^2 = \begin{cases} \Delta_{2\left(\frac{n_2'+1}{2}\right)}^2 & \text{if } n_2' \text{ is odd} \\[2ex] \Delta_{2\left(\frac{n_2'}{2}\right)}^2 + \Delta_{2\left(\frac{n_2'+2}{2}\right)}^2 & \text{if } n_2' \text{ is even} \end{cases}$$

where   □

Remark 3.6 The median RSS should be preferred to RSS whenever.

$$E\left(\sum_{j=1}^{n_2'} \Delta_{2(j)}^2\right) > E\left(\frac{\Delta_{2(m)}^2}{2}\right)$$

                                                                                            □

3.4 The Estimation of a Difference

Bouza (1983) considered the estimation of the difference of population means with missing observations. We use the considerations of Pi-Ehr (1971) that the population can be stratified as follows $U = U_1 \cup U_2 \cup U_3$, $U_j \cap U_j = \emptyset, \forall i \neq j'$, $j,j' = 1,2,3$.

A SRSWR sample s is selected from U for estimating $D = \mu_X - \mu_Y$. The units in s can be denoted as $s = s_1 \cup s_2 \cup s_3$, $s_j \cup \cap s_{j'}, \forall i \neq j', j,j' = 1,2,3$. The sample size is $|s| = n$. The units in s_1 give information on X and Y, but we have missing information of Y those in s_2 and in X by the respondents in s_3. Without loosing in generality we may rearrange the units in s and to denote:

$$s_1 = \{i \in s | 1 \leq i \leq n_1\}, /s_1/ = n_1$$
$$s_2 = \{1 \in s | n_1 + 1 \leq i \leq n_1 + n_2\}, /s_2/ = n_2$$
$$s_3 = \{i \in s | n_1 + n_2 + 1 \leq i \leq n\}, /s_1/ = n_3$$

The need of obtaining information from the non-respondents establishes that the subsamples s_j, $j = 2,3$, should be resampled for obtaining it. This decision is reasonable when we expect that the means and variances of the variables in the strata are very different. Denote by $s'_j \subset s_j$ the corresponding subsample of *size* $|s'_j| = n'_j$, $j = 2,3$. Using the notation of Bouza and Prabhu-Ajgaonkar (1993) each subsample s_t belongs to a stratum U_t, $t = 1, 2, 3$. The information provided by s permits to calculate

$$\bar{x}_1 = \frac{\sum_{i=1}^{n_1} x_i}{n_1}, \bar{y}_1 = \frac{\sum_{i=1}^{n_1} y_i}{n_1}, \bar{d}_1 = \frac{\sum_{i=1}^{n_1} (x_i - y_i)}{n_1} = \frac{\sum_{i=1}^{n_1} d_i}{n_1}, \bar{x}_2 = \frac{\sum_{i=n_1+1}^{n_1+n_2} x_i}{n_2}, \bar{y}_3 = \frac{\sum_{i=n_1+n_2+1}^{n} y_i}{n_3}$$

An unbiased estimator of the difference between the population means is

$$d_{srs} = \bar{\bar{x}}^* - \bar{\bar{y}}^*$$

where

$$\bar{\bar{x}}^* = \frac{\sum_{t\in\{1,2\}} n_t\bar{x}_t + n_3\bar{x}_3'}{n} = \sum_{t\in\{1,2\}} w_t\bar{x}_t + w_3\bar{x}_3'$$

$$\bar{\bar{y}}^* = \frac{\sum_{t\in\{1,3\}} n_t\bar{y}_t + n_2\bar{y}_2'}{n} = \sum_{t\in\{1,3\}} w_t\bar{y}_t + w_3\bar{y}_2'$$

where

$$\bar{x}_3' = \frac{\sum_{i=n_1+n_2+1}^{n} x_i}{n_3'}, \bar{y}_2' = \frac{\sum_{i=n_1+1}^{n_1+n_2} y_i}{n_2'}$$

and

$$w_i = \frac{n_i}{n}$$

The corresponding model is characterized in the following proposition.

Theorem 3.7 (Bouza and Prabhu-Ajgaonkar 1993). *Take a SRSWR-sample selected from U. The units in the stratum U_1 report X and Y, the units in U_2 only report X while Y is the variable reported by U_3 at the first visit. The estimator*

$$d_{srs} = \bar{\bar{x}}^* - \bar{\bar{y}}^*$$

is unbiased for D and its expected error is

$$\overline{V} = V_1 = \frac{\sigma_d^2 + \varpi_2\sigma_{Y(2)}^2 + \varpi_3\sigma_{X(3)}^2}{n}$$

$$W_i = \frac{N_i}{N} = \frac{\text{number of units in } U_i}{N} \text{ and } N = N_1 + N_2 + N_3$$

and ϖ_i, $i = 2,3$ is the coefficient generated by the subsampling rule. ☐

Let us take r as fixed, $n_j = rm_j$, then the subsampling size among the non-respondents of stratum U_j. As $n'_j = rm'_j = \theta rm_j$. It makes sense to use as concomitant variable X (Y) if $j = 2(3)$. Considering the conditional unbiasedness of

$$\bar{z}'_{\text{jrss}} = \frac{\sum\limits_{t=1}^{r}\sum\limits_{i=1}^{m'_j} z_{(i:m'_j)t}}{rm'_j}, j = 2(3), \quad \text{if } Z = Y(X)$$

Mimicking the structure of d_{srs} we consider the estimator.

$$\bar{d}_{\text{rss}} = w_1 d_{\text{1rss}} + w_2\left(\bar{x}_{\text{2rss}} - \bar{y}'_{\text{2rss}}\right) + w_3\left(\bar{x}'_{\text{3rss}} - \bar{y}_{\text{3rss}}\right), \ d_{\text{1rss}} = \sum\limits_{i=1}^{m_1}\sum\limits_{t=1}^{r}\frac{d_{(i:m)t}}{n_1}$$

The use of RSS instead of SRSWR was studied by Bouza (2002). The corresponding results are given in the following proposition.

Proposition 3.8 *Take a RSS-sample selected from U. The units in the stratum U_1 report X and Y, the units in U_2 only report X while Y is the variable reported by U_3 at the first visit. An unbiased estimator of the difference of the means is*

$$\bar{d}_{\text{rss}} = w_1 d_{\text{1rss}} + w_2\left(\bar{x}_{\text{2rss}} - \bar{y}'_{\text{2rss}}\right) + w_3\left(\bar{x}'_{\text{3rss}} - \bar{y}_{\text{3rss}}\right) w_i = \frac{n_i}{n}$$

and its error is

$$EV\left(\bar{d}_{\text{rss}}|s\right) = \frac{\sigma_d^2}{n} + \frac{\varpi\sigma_{2Y}^2}{n} + \frac{\varpi\sigma_{3X}^2}{n} - \left(\frac{\Delta_d^2}{n} + \Psi\right),$$

$$\Psi = E\left(\frac{\sum\limits_{i=1}^{m_2} W_2\Delta_{2Y(i:m_2)}^2}{\upsilon m_2} + \frac{\sum\limits_{i=1}^{m_3} W_3\Delta_{3X(i:m_3)}^2}{\upsilon m_3}\right)$$

Proof Take

$$\bar{d}_{\text{rss}} = w_1 d_{\text{1rss}} + \sum\limits_{j=2}^{3} w_j\left(\bar{x}_{\text{jrss}} - \bar{y}_{\text{jrss}}\right) + w_2\left(\bar{x}_{\text{2rss}} - \bar{y}'_{\text{2rs}}\right) + w_3\left(\bar{x}'_{\text{3rss}} - \bar{y}_3\right)$$

The sum of the two first terms of $\bar{d}_{\text{rss}}$ is equal to d_{rss}, hence the conditional variance with expectation equal to $\bar{V} = V_1 = \frac{\sigma_d^2 + \varpi_2\sigma_{Y(2)}^2 + \varpi_3\sigma_{X(3)}^2}{n}$. Let us analyze the second term.

$$V\left(\bar{y}_{\text{2rss}} - \bar{y}'_{\text{2rss}}|s\right) = E\left(\bar{y}_{\text{2rss}} - \bar{y}_{\text{2rss}}|s\right)^2 - V\left(\bar{y}_{\text{2rss}}|s\right)$$

because

$$\bar{y}_{\text{2rss}} - \mu_{2Y} = \left(\bar{y}'_{\text{2rss}} - \bar{y}_{\text{2rss}}\right) + \left(\bar{y}_{\text{2rss}} - \mu_{2Y}\right)$$

The cross expectation's expected value is zero. In this case, the RSS is balanced and we may express the variance of the os as a function of the variance of Y in U_2 and the gains in accuracy measured by the $\Delta_{2Y(i)}^2$'s as

$$V\left(\bar{y}_2 - \bar{y}'_{2rss}\middle|s\right) = \sigma^2_{Y(2)}\left(\frac{1}{n'_2} - \frac{1}{n_2}\right) - \sum_{i=1}^{m_2}\frac{\Delta^2_{2Y(i)}}{n'_2 m_2}$$

substituting $n'_2 = \theta r m_2$ we obtain:

$$V\left(\bar{y}_{2rss} - \bar{y}'_{2rss}\middle|s\right) = \frac{\sigma^2_{Y(2)}}{n_2}\left(\frac{1-\theta}{\theta}\right) - \sum_{i=1}^{m_2}\frac{\Delta^2_{2Y(i:m_2)}}{\theta m n_2} = V_2$$

A similar reasoning with the last term yields

$$V\left(\bar{x}'_{3rss} - \bar{y}_{3rss}\middle|s\right) = \frac{\sigma^2_{X(3)}}{n_3}\left(\frac{1-\theta}{\theta}\right) - \sum_{i=1}^{m_2}\frac{\Delta^2_{3X(i:m_3)}}{\theta m n_3} = V_3$$

$$V\left(\bar{d}_{rss}\middle|s\right) = V_1 + w_2^2 V_2 + w_3^2 V_3$$

Now we have that as n_j is a Binomial random variable with expectation $nW_j = nN_j/N$

$$V\left(\bar{d}_{rss}\middle|s\right) = V_1 + w_2^2 V_2 + w_3^2 V_3$$

and

$$EV\left(\bar{d}_{rss}\middle|s\right) = \frac{\sigma^2_d}{n} + \frac{\varpi\sigma^2_{2Y}}{n} + \frac{\varpi\sigma^2_{3X}}{n} - \left(\frac{\Delta^2_d}{n} + \Psi\right)$$

where

$$\Psi = E\left(\frac{\sum_{i=1}^{m_2}\Delta^2_{2Y(i:m_2)}}{\upsilon m_2} + \frac{\sum_{i=1}^{m_3}\Delta^2_{3X(i:m_3)}}{\upsilon m_3}\right)$$

$\square$

Remark 3.9 The last term of the expected error is always positive and represents the gain in accuracy due to RSS. Hence the use of RSS for subsampling the *NR* when *D* is estimated is a better alternative than the *SRSWR* strategy. $\square$

3.5 Product-Type Estimators

Bouza (2008) analyzed the use of RSS alternatives when a product estimator is used. The product estimator is defined by

$$\bar{y}_p = \frac{\bar{x}\bar{y}}{\mu_X}$$

where

$$\bar{z} = \frac{\sum_{i=1}^{n} z_j}{n}; z = x, y, \quad \mu_X = \frac{\sum_{i=1}^{N} X_j}{N}$$

It is closely related to ratio estimators, see Cocrhan (1977), David-Sukhatme (1974). Its expectation is given by

$$E(\bar{y}_p) = \frac{E(\overline{xy})}{\mu_X \mu_Y} = \mu_Y + \frac{\sigma_{XY}}{n\bar{X}}$$

$$\text{where } \sigma_{XY} = \frac{\sum_{i=1}^{N}(X_j - \mu_X)(Y_j - \mu_Y)}{N}; \quad \mu_Y = \frac{\sum_{i=1}^{N} X_j}{N}$$

Hence it has a bias $B(\bar{y}_p) = \frac{\sigma_{XY}}{n\mu_X}$. Its variance is

$$V(\bar{y}_p) = \frac{\sigma_Y^2 + R^2 \sigma_X^2 + 2R\sigma_{XY}}{N}$$

where

$$R = \frac{\mu_Y}{\mu_X}, \sigma_Z^2 = \frac{\sum_{j=1}^{N}(Z_j - \mu_Z)^2}{N}, Z = X, Y$$

A version of it is

$$\bar{y}_{p*} = \frac{\sum_{i=1}^{n} x_j y_j}{n\mu_X}$$

and it has the same bias and variance as $\bar{y}_p$.

These estimators can be used for deriving the estimation of the mean of the NR stratum.

Agrawal and Sthapit (1997) derived the exact formulas for the bias and variance of the product estimator under simple random sampling. Its asymptotic normality was rigorously established under weak and interpretable regularity conditions on the finite populations.

Let us consider the separate product estimator

$$\bar{y}_{ps} = \frac{n_1 \bar{y}_1 + n_2 \bar{y}'_{2p}}{n} = \frac{n_1 \bar{y}_1 + n_2 \bar{y}_2}{n} + \frac{n_2(\bar{y}'_{2p} - \bar{y}_2)}{n}$$

where

$$\bar{y}'_{2p} = \frac{\bar{y}'_2 \bar{x}_2}{\mu_X}$$

The first member at the right-hand side of $\bar{y}_{ps}$ is the mean of Y in s. Hence the bias of $\bar{y}_{ps}$ depends on the expectation of the last term. The conditional expectation of it, for a fixed n'_2, is equal to the product estimator based on the subsample s_2. Therefore

$$E\left(\frac{n_2(\bar{y}'_{2p} - \bar{y}_2)}{n}\,\Big|n'_2\right) = \frac{n_2\bar{y}_2\bar{x}_2}{n\mu_X} - \frac{n_2\bar{y}_2}{n}$$

as

$$E\left(\frac{n_2\bar{y}_2\bar{x}_2}{n\mu_X} - \frac{n_2\bar{y}_2}{n}\,\Big|n_2\right) = \frac{n_2}{n}\left(\frac{\sigma_{2XY}}{n_2\mu_X}\right),$$

where

$$\sigma_{2XY} = \frac{\sum_{j=1}^{N_2}(X_{2j} - \mu_{2X})(Y_{2j} - \mu_{2Y})}{N_2}, \ \mu_{Z(2)} = \frac{\sum_{j=1}^{N_2}Z_{2j}}{N_2}, \ Z = X, Y$$

Then the bias is equal to

$$B_{ps} = B(\bar{y}_{ps}) = \frac{\sigma_{XY}}{n\mu_X}$$

Using the results obtained previously we have that under the regularity condition

$$R1: \frac{\sigma_{2ZY}}{n'_2\mu_{2Y}\mu_X} \cong \frac{\sum_{j=1}^{n_2}(y_{2j} - \bar{y}_2)(x_{2j} - \bar{x}_2)}{n'_2\mu_{2Y}\mu_X}$$

we have that

$$E\left(E\left(\bar{y}_{ps}\,|n'_2\right)\,|n_2\right) \cong \bar{y} + \frac{\mu_{Y2}\rho_{2XY}C_{2Y}C_{2X}}{\theta n}$$

The variance of $\bar{y}_{ps}$ is obtained by calculating

$$V\left(E\left(E\left(\bar{y}_{ps}\,|n'_2, n_e\right)\right)\right) + E\left(V\left(E\left(\bar{y}_{ps}\,|n'_2, n_e\right)\right)\right) + E\left(E\left(V\left(\bar{y}_{ps}\,|n'_2, n_e\right)\right)\right)$$

Let us compute the first term

$$V\left(E\left(E\left(\bar{y}_{ps}\,|n'_2, n_2\right)\right)\right) = V\left(\bar{y} + \frac{C_{2X}C_{2Y}\mu_{2Y}}{n}\right)$$

$$= V(\bar{y}) + V\left(\frac{C_{2X}C_{2Y}\mu_{2Y}}{\vartheta n}\right) + 2\mathrm{Cov}\left(\bar{y}, \frac{C_{2X}C_{2Y}\mu_{2Y}}{n}\right)$$

The first term is the variance of the sample mean in SRSWR

$$V(\bar{y}) = \frac{\sigma_Y^2}{n}$$

while the second and third ones are equal to zero.

For the second term we have the expression

$$E\big(V\big(E(\bar{y}_{ps}|n_2')|n_2\big)\big) = E\left(V\left(\bar{y} + \frac{n_2}{n}(\bar{y}_{2p} - \bar{y}_2)|n_2\right)\right)$$
$$= E\left(\left(\frac{n_2}{n}\right)^2 V\big((\bar{y}_{2p} - \bar{y}_2)|n_2\big)\right)$$

Calculating the conditional variance we obtain

$$V\big((\bar{y}_{2p} - \bar{y}_2)|n_2\big) = V\big((\bar{y}_{2p})|n_2\big) + V\big((\bar{y}_2)|n_2\big)$$
$$- 2\mathrm{Cov}\big((\bar{y}_{2p}, \bar{y}_2)|n_2\big)$$

The first two terms are easily derived as

$$V\big((\bar{y}_{2p})|n_2\big) \cong \frac{\sigma_{2Y}^2 + R_2^2\sigma_{2X}^2 + 2R_2\sigma_{2XY}}{n_2}, \quad V\big((\bar{y}_2)|n_2\big) = \frac{\sigma_{2Y}^2}{n_2}$$

For computing the third term we relay on the properties of the sampling moments enounced by David and Sukhatme (1974). This term can be written as

$$\mathrm{Cov}\big((\bar{y}_{2p}, \bar{y}_2)|n_2\big) = E\left(\frac{\bar{y}_2^2\bar{x}_2}{\mu_X}|n_2\right) - \left(\mu_{Y(2)} + \frac{\mu_{Y(2)}\rho_2 C_{2X}C_{2Y}}{n_2}\right)\mu_{Y(2)}$$

As

$$E\big(\bar{y}_2^2\bar{x}_2|n_2\big) = \mu_{Y(2)}^2\mu_{X(2)} + \frac{2\mu_{Y(2)}\sigma_{2XY} + \mu_X\sigma_Y^2}{n_2} + O(n^{-2})$$

we have that

$$\mathrm{Cov}\big((\bar{y}_{2p}, \bar{y}_2)|n_2\big) \cong \frac{\mu_{Y(2)}^2}{\mu_X}\left(\mu_{X(2)} - \frac{\rho_2 C_{2X}C_{2Y}}{n_2}\right) + \frac{2\mu_{Y(2)}\sigma_{2XY} +}{n_2\mu_X}$$
$$+ \frac{\sigma_{Y(2)}^2 - \mu_{Y(2)}^2}{n_2}$$

Substituting the terms derived previously we have that

$$V\big((\bar{y}_{2p} - \bar{y}_2)|n_2\big) \cong \frac{R_2^2\sigma_{2X}^2 + 2\sigma_{2XY}\left(R_2 - \frac{2\mu_{Y(2)}}{\mu_{X(2)}}\right)}{n_2}$$
$$- 2\left(\frac{\mu_{Y(2)}^2}{\mu_X}\left(\mu_{X(2)} - \frac{\rho_2 C_{2X}C_{2Y}}{n_2}\right) - \frac{\mu_{Y(2)}^2}{n_2}\right)$$

The analyzed variance term is derived by computing the unconditional expectation

$$E\left(\left(\frac{n_2}{n}\right)^2 V\left((\bar{y}_{2p} - \bar{y}_2)|n_2\right)\right) \cong W_2(S(1) + S(2)) - 2\lambda_{2XY}$$

where

$$S(1) = \frac{R_2^2 \sigma_{X(2)}^2 + 2\sigma_{2XY}\left(R_2 - \frac{2\mu_{Y(2)}}{\mu_{2X}}\right)}{n}$$

$$S(2) = 2\left(\frac{\rho_2 C_{2X} C_{2Y}}{n\mu_X} + \frac{\mu_{Y(2)}^2}{n\mu_X}\right)$$

and

$$\lambda_{2XY} = \left(\frac{\mu_{Y(2)}^2 \mu_{X(2)}}{n\mu_X}\right)(nW_2^2 + nW_1 W_2)$$

The third term of the sampling error is

$$E\left(E\left(V(\bar{y}_{ps}|n_2')|n_2\right)\right) = E\left(E\left(\left(\frac{n_2}{n}\right)^2 E\left(\left(\bar{y}_{2p}' - \bar{y}_2\right)^2 |n_2'\right)|n_2\right)\right)$$

As $\bar{y}_{2p}' - \mu_{Y(2)} = \left(\bar{y}_{2p}' - \bar{y}_2\right) + \left(\bar{y}_2 - \mu_{Y(2)}\right)$ is derived that

$$E\left(\left(\bar{y}_{2p}' - \bar{y}_2\right)^2 |n_2'\right) = E\left(\left(\bar{y}_2 - \mu_{Y(2)}\right)^2 |n_2'\right) - E\left(\left(\bar{y}_2 - \mu_{Y(2)}\right)^2 |n_2'\right)$$

$$= \frac{(1 - \theta)\sigma_{Y(2)}^2}{\theta n_2}$$

because the expectation of the cross term is equal to zero. As a consequence

$$E\left(E\left(V(\bar{y}_{ps}|n_2')|n_2\right)\right) = \frac{W_2(1 - \theta)\sigma_{Y(2)}^2}{n\theta}$$

these results enhance to give a characterization of the proposed estimator.

Proposition 3.9 $\bar{y}_{ps}$ *is asymptotically unbiased as an estimator of the population mean and its variance is*

$$V(\bar{y}_{ps}) = \frac{\sigma_Y^2}{n} + \frac{W_2 \sigma_{ps(2)}}{n} + \frac{W_2(1 - \theta)\sigma_{Y(2)}^2}{n\theta} - 2\lambda_{2XY}^*$$

where

$$\sigma_{ps(2)} \cong R_2^2\sigma_{2X}^2 + 2\sigma_{2XY}\left(R_2 - \frac{2\mu_{Y(2)}}{\mu_{2X}}\right) + \left(2\left(\frac{\rho_2 C_{2X}C_{2Y}}{\mu_X} + \frac{\mu_{Y(2)}^2}{\mu_X}\right)\right)$$

$$\lambda_{2XY}^* = \left(\frac{\mu_{2(2)Y}^2\mu_{X(2)}}{\mu_X}\right)$$

if the regularity condition R1 holds.

Proof The first result is derived by fixing that $\lim_{n\to\infty}\left(\frac{\sigma_{2XY}}{n\mu_X}\right) = 0$. The expression of the variance is obtained by summing $V(\bar{y})$, $E\left(\left(\frac{n_2}{n}\right)^2 V\left((\bar{y}_{2p} - \bar{y}_2)|n_2\right)\right)$ and $E\left(\left(\bar{y}_{2p}' - \bar{y}_2\right)^2 |n_2'\right)$ and doing some algebraic work. □

A combined product estimator of μ_Y for non-responses is the alternative the estimator

$$\bar{y}_{pc} = \left(\frac{n_1\bar{y}_1 + n_2\bar{y}_2'}{n}\right)\frac{\bar{x}}{\mu_x}$$

It uses the combination of the subsamples. As stated previously

$$\bar{y}_{pc} = \left(\frac{n_1\bar{y}_1 + n_2\bar{y}_2}{n}\right)\frac{\bar{x}}{\mu_x} + \left(\frac{n_2(\bar{y}_2' - \bar{y}_2)}{n}\right)\frac{\bar{x}}{\mu_x}$$

The first term is the expression of the product estimator in the original sample. The conditional expectation of the second term is zero. Hence we have that $\bar{y}_{pc}$ is asymptotically unbiased because

$$EEE\left(\bar{y}_{pc}|n_2', n_2\right) = E(\bar{y}_p) = \mu_Y + \mu_Y\left(\frac{\rho C_X C_Y}{n}\right)$$

and the last term (the bias) tends to zero for large sample size values.
The unconditional variance of $\bar{y}_{pc}$ is given by

$$V\left(EE\left(\bar{y}_{pc}|n_2', n_2\right)\right) = V(\bar{y}_p) = \frac{\sigma_Y^2 + R^2\sigma_X^2 + 2R\sigma_{XY}}{n} = V(1)$$

It is easily derived that

$$E\left(V(E(\bar{y}_{pc}|n_2')|n_2)\right) = E(V(\bar{y}_p|n_2) = 0$$

because at the second conditional level we are calculating the variance of a constant.

Let us calculate the last component of the sampling error. Using the result derived for $E\left(\left(\frac{n_2}{n}\right)^2 V\left((\bar{y}_{2p} - \bar{y}_2)|n_2\right)\right)$ we have that

$$V(\bar{y}_{pc}|n_2') = \left(\frac{n_2\bar{x}}{n\mu_x}\right)^2 E\left((\bar{y}_2' - \bar{y}_2)^2|n_2'\right) = \left(\frac{n_2\bar{x}}{n\mu_x}\right)^2 \frac{(1-\theta)\sigma_{2Y}^2}{\theta n_2}$$

The expectation conditional to a fixed n_2 is

$$E\left(\left(\frac{n_1\bar{x}_1 + n_2\bar{x}_2}{n}\right)^2 | n_2\right) = \left(\frac{n_1}{n}\right)^2 \left(\mu_{X(1)}^2 + \frac{\sigma_{X(1)}^2}{n_1}\right) + \left(\frac{n_2}{n}\right)^2 \left(\mu_{X(2)}^2 + \frac{\sigma_{X(2)}^2}{n_2}\right)$$
$$+ 2\left(\frac{n_1 n_2}{n^2}\right)\left(\mu_{X(1)}\mu_{X(2)}\right)$$

Calculating $E(n_i^2)$, $I = 1, 2$, $E(n_1 n_2)$, and adding this result to $V(1)$, after grouping we obtain

$$V(\bar{y}_{pc}) = \frac{\sigma_Y^2 + R^2\sigma_X^2 + 2R\sigma_{XY}}{n}$$
$$+ \frac{(1-\theta)\sigma_{Y(2)}^2}{\theta\mu_X^2}\left(\mu_X^2 + \frac{W_1 W_2\left(\mu_{X(1)} - \mu_{X(2)}\right)^2}{n} + \frac{\sum_{i=1}^2 W_i\sigma_{X(i)}^2}{n}\right)$$

Then we have the following Lemma.

Proposition 3.10 *The estimator of* μ_Y. $\bar{y}_{pc}$ *is asymptotically unbiased and its variance is given by*

$$V(\bar{y}_{pc}) = \frac{\sigma_Y^2 + R^2\sigma_X^2 + 2R\sigma_{XY}}{n}$$
$$+ \frac{(1-\theta)\sigma_{Y(2)}^2}{\theta\mu_X^2}\left(\mu_X^2 + \frac{W_1 W_2\left(\mu_{X(1)} - \mu_{X(2)}\right)^2}{n} + \frac{\sum_{i=1}^2 W_i\sigma_{X(i)}^2}{n}\right)$$

$\square$

3.6 The Non-response Problem: Double Sampling

We will consider that double sampling is used for obtaining a sample $s*$ from U using SRSWR. This is the basic procedure used in textbooks, see Cochran (1977), Sing Deo (2003), and in many approaches to the study of NR, see for example Singh-Kumar (2008a), Bouza (2011).: A cheap variable X, correlated with Y, is measured in the n* units selected. We are able to compute the means of the first stage and second stage samples of X : $\bar{x}_{s*} = \frac{\sum_{i=1}^{n*} x_i}{n*}$ and $\bar{x} = \frac{\sum_{i=1}^n x_i}{n}$.

Non-responses are present in the second stage sample and a subsample among the non-respondents is selected. Singh-Kumar (2009) considered this problem for simple random sampling. They proposed the family of estimators characterized by

$$\bar{y}^* = \bar{\bar{y}}\left(\frac{a\bar{\bar{x}}+b}{a\bar{x}_{s^*}+b}\right)^{\alpha}\left(\frac{a\bar{x}+b}{a\bar{x}_{s^*}+b}\right)^{\beta}$$

The sampler fixes the constants α and β as well as a and b. They can be constants or functions, a different from zero. Taking

$$\varepsilon = \frac{\bar{\bar{y}}-\mu_Y}{\mu_Y}, \theta = \frac{\bar{\bar{x}}-\mu_X}{\mu_X}, \vartheta = \frac{\bar{x}_{s^*}-\mu_X}{\mu_X}, \omega = \frac{\bar{x}-\mu_X}{\mu_X}$$

Theorem 3.11 (Singh-Kumar 2009). *The bias of*

$$\bar{y}^* = \bar{\bar{y}}\left(\frac{a\bar{\bar{x}}+b}{a\bar{x}_{s^*}+b}\right)^{\alpha}\left(\frac{a\bar{x}+b}{a\bar{x}_{s^*}+b}\right)^{\beta}$$

is $B(\bar{y}^*) = \mu_Y(\varphi_1 + \varphi_2)$ defining

$$\varphi_1 = \left(\gamma\phi\left[\alpha K_{xy} + \frac{\alpha-1}{2}\phi\right] + \beta\left(K_{xy} + \alpha\phi + \frac{\beta-1}{2}\phi\right)\right)c_x^2$$

$$\varphi_2 = \lambda\alpha\phi\left(K_{x_2y} + \frac{\alpha-1}{2}\phi\right)c_{x_2}^2$$

where $\gamma = \frac{1}{n} - \frac{1}{n^*}, \lambda = \frac{W_2(K-1)}{n}, c_x^2 = \frac{\sigma_x^2}{\mu_x^2}, c_{x_2}^2 = \frac{\sigma_{x_2}^2}{\mu_{x_2}^2}, K_{xy} = \frac{\mu_x\sigma_{xy}}{\mu_y\sigma_x^2}, K_{x_2y} = \frac{\mu_{x_2}\sigma_{x_2y}^2}{\mu_y\sigma_{x_2}^2 x_2}$

$$\sigma_{xy} = E(X-\mu_x)(Y-\mu_Y), \sigma_{x_2y} = E((X-\mu_x)(Y-\mu_Y)/U_2)$$

The variance is given by

$$V(\bar{\bar{y}}^*) = \mu_Y^2(\delta_1 + \delta_2)$$

defining

$$\delta_1 = \left(\gamma\left[c_Y^2 + (\alpha+\beta)\phi((\alpha+\beta)\phi + 2K_{xy})c_x^2\right]\right)$$

$$\delta_2 = \lambda\left(c_{y_2}^2 + \alpha\phi(\alpha\phi + 2K_{x_2y})c_{x_2}^2\right) + \frac{c_y^2}{n^*}$$

$$, c_y^2 = \frac{\sigma_y^2}{\mu_y^2}, c_{y_2}^2 = \frac{\sigma_{y_2}^2}{\mu_{y_2}^2},$$

□

We are going to derive the RSS counter part of this family. The first phase sample is selected using SRSWR and the information on X is used for selecting the initial sample and to subsample the non-respondents. Our proposal is to use

$$\bar{y}^*_{\text{rss}} = \bar{\bar{y}}_{\text{rss}} \left(\frac{a\bar{\bar{x}}_{\text{rss}} + b}{a\bar{x}_{s^*} + b} \right)^\alpha \left(\frac{a\bar{x}_{\text{rss}} + b}{a\bar{x}_{s^*} + b} \right)^\beta$$

Hence

$$\varepsilon_{\text{rss}} = \frac{\bar{\bar{y}}_{\text{rss}} - \mu_Y}{\mu_Y}, \theta_{\text{rss}} = \frac{\bar{\bar{x}}_{\text{rss}} - \mu_X}{\mu_X}, \vartheta = \frac{\bar{x}_{s^*} - \mu_X}{\mu_X}, \omega_{\text{rss}} = \frac{\bar{x}_{\text{rss}} - \mu_X}{\mu_X}$$

Let us represent the involved estimators by

$$\bar{\bar{y}}_{\text{rss}} = \mu_Y(1 + \varepsilon_{\text{rss}})$$
$$\bar{\bar{x}}_{\text{rss}} = \mu_X(1 + \theta_{\text{rss}})$$
$$\bar{x}_{s^*} = \mu_X(1 + \vartheta)$$
$$\bar{x}_{\text{rss}} = \mu_X(1 + \omega_{\text{rss}})$$

Due to the unbiasedness of the estimators $E(Z) = 0, Z = \varepsilon_{\text{rss}}, \theta_{\text{rss}}, \vartheta, \omega_{\text{rss}}$. Taking $\phi = \frac{a\mu_X}{a\mu_x + b}$ we can rewrite $\bar{y}^*_{\text{rss}}$ as

$$\bar{\bar{y}}^*_{\text{rss}} = \mu_Y \left[(1 + \varepsilon_{\text{rss}})(1 + \phi\theta_{\text{rss}})^\alpha (1 + \phi\vartheta)^{-\alpha}(1 + \phi\omega_{\text{rss}})^\beta (1 + \phi\vartheta)^{-\beta} \right]$$

Note that

$$E(\varepsilon_{\text{rss}})^2 = \frac{E(\bar{\bar{y}}_{\text{rss}} - \mu_Y)^2}{\mu_Y^2} = \frac{\frac{\sigma_Y^2}{n} + \frac{W_2(K-1)\sigma_{2Y}^2}{n^*}}{\mu_Y^2} - \frac{W_2(K-1)E\left(\frac{\sum_{i=1}^{m_2} \Delta_{2Y(i:m_2)}^2}{m_2} \right)}{\mu_Y^2}$$

$$E(\theta_{\text{rss}})^2 = \frac{\frac{\sigma_x^2}{n} + \frac{W_2(K-1)\sigma_{2x}^2}{n}}{\mu_x^2} - \frac{W_2(K-1)E\left(\frac{\sum_{i=1}^{m_2} \Delta_{2x(i:m_2)}^2}{nm_2} \right)}{\mu_x^2}$$

$$E(\vartheta)^2 = \frac{E(\bar{x}_{s^*} - \mu_X)^2}{\mu_X^2} = \frac{\sigma_X^2}{n^* \mu_X^2}$$

$$E(\omega_{\text{rss}})^2 = \frac{\frac{\sigma_x^2}{n} - \frac{\sum_{i=1}^{m} \Delta_{x(i)}^2}{rn}}{\mu_x^2}$$

Under the hypothesis $|\phi Z| < 1$, $/\phi Z/ < 1, Z = \varepsilon_{\text{rss}}, \theta_{\text{rss}}, \vartheta, \omega_{\text{rss}}$, an expansion in Taylor Series of $\bar{\bar{y}}^*_{\text{rss}}$ may be worked out. Grouping conveniently the terms we have that

$$\bar{\bar{y}}^*_{\text{rss}} - \mu_Y \cong D(1)$$

$$= \mu_Y \Big[\varepsilon_{\text{rss}} + \beta(\omega_{\text{rss}} + \varepsilon_{\text{rss}}\omega_{\text{rss}} - \varepsilon_{\text{rss}}\vartheta) + \alpha\phi(\theta_{\text{rss}} + \varepsilon_{\text{rss}}\theta_{\text{rss}} - \varepsilon_{\text{rss}}\vartheta)$$

$$- (\alpha + \beta)\phi\vartheta + \alpha\beta\phi^2 \left(\vartheta^2 + \vartheta(\omega_{\text{rss}} + \theta_{\text{rss}}) + \vartheta\omega_{\text{rss}}\right) - \phi^2 \left(\beta^2\vartheta\omega_{\text{rss}} + \alpha^2\vartheta\theta_{\text{rss}}\right)$$

$$+ \frac{\beta(\beta + 1)\phi^2}{2}\left(\vartheta^2 + \omega^2_{\text{rss}}\right) + \frac{\alpha(\alpha + 1)\phi^2}{2}\left(\vartheta^2 + \omega^2_{\text{rss}}\right) \Big]$$

Note that the cross products are expressed by the general expression

$$\sum_{i=1}^{h} \left(Z_{(i)} - \mu_{Z_{(i)}}\right)\left(Z'_{(i)} - \mu_{Z'_{(i)}}\right) = \sum_{i=1}^{h} \left(Z_{(i)} \mp \mu_Z - \mu_{Z_{(i)}}\right)\left(Z'_{(i)} \mp \mu_{Z'} - \mu_{Z'_{(i)}}\right)$$

$$= \sum_{i=1}^{h}\left(Z_{(i)} - \mu_Z\right)\left(Z'_{(i)} - \mu_{Z'}\right) - \sum_{i=1}^{h} Z_{(i)}\Delta_{Z'_{(i)}} + Z'_{(i)}\Delta_{Z_{(i)}} - \Delta_{Z_{(i)}}\Delta_{Z'_{(i)}}$$

$$= (h - 1)(\sigma_{ZZ'} + \Psi_{ZZ'})$$

On the other hand, the conditional expectations of the RSS estimators are

$$E(\bar{x}_{\text{rss}}/s^*) = E\big(E(\bar{\bar{x}}_{\text{rss}}/s)/s^*\big) = \bar{x}^*$$

Using these results we have that

$$E(\varepsilon_{\text{rss}}\theta_{\text{rss}}) = \frac{\sigma_{XY} + \Psi_{XY}}{n\mu_x\mu_y} + \frac{W_2(K - 1)(\sigma_{X_2Y} + \Psi_{X_2Y})}{n\mu_x\mu_y}$$

$$E(\varepsilon_{\text{rss}}\vartheta) = \frac{\sigma_{XY} + \Psi_{XY}}{n^*\mu_x\mu_y}$$

$$E(\varepsilon_{\text{rss}}\omega_{\text{rss}}) = \frac{\sigma_{XY} + \Psi_{XY}}{n\mu_x\mu_y}$$

defining

$$\Psi_{X_2Y} = -E\left(\frac{\sum_{i=1}^{m'_2} X_{(i)2}\Delta_{x_{(i)2}} + Y_{(i)2}\Delta_{y_{(i)2}} - \Delta_{x_{(i)2}}\Delta_{y_{(i)}}}{m_2}\right)$$

$$\Psi_{XY} = -E\left(\frac{\sum_{i=1}^{m} X_{(i)}\Delta_{x_{(i)}} + Y_{(i)}\Delta_{y_{(i)}} - \Delta_{x_{(i)}}\Delta_{y_{(i)}}}{m}\right)$$

In addition

$$E(\omega_{\text{rss}}\theta_{\text{rss}}) = \frac{\sigma^2_x + x}{n\mu^2_x}, \quad \Psi_X = -\frac{\sum_{i=1}^{m} \Delta^2_{x_{(8i)}}}{r}$$

$$E(\vartheta\theta_{\mathrm{rss}}) = \frac{\sigma_x^2}{n^*\mu_x^2}$$

$$E(\vartheta\omega_{\mathrm{rss}}) = \frac{\sigma_x^2}{n^*\mu_x^2}$$

Substituting in $D(1)$ after some algebraic work we obtain that the bias of $\bar{y}_{\mathrm{rss}}^*$ is

$$B(\bar{y}_{\mathrm{rss}}^*) = \mu_Y(\varphi_{1\mathrm{rss}} + \varphi_{2\mathrm{rss}})$$

$$\varphi_{1\mathrm{rss}} = \left(\gamma\phi\left[\alpha\left(K_{xy}c_x^2 + \frac{XY}{n\mu_x\mu_y}\right) + \frac{\alpha-1}{2}\phi\left(c_x^2 + \frac{X}{n\mu_x^2}\right)\right]\right.$$

$$\left. + \beta\left(K_{xy}c_x^2 + \frac{\Psi_{XY}}{n\mu_x\mu_y} + \alpha\phi\left(c_x^2 + \frac{\Psi_X}{n\mu_x^2}\right) + \frac{\beta-1}{2}\phi c_x^2\right)\right)$$

$$\Psi_{z2} = -\frac{E\left(\frac{\sum_{i=1}^{m_2}\Delta_{2z(i:m_2)}^2}{m_2}\right)}{n\mu_z^2}, z = x, y$$

For a large value of n the bias tends to zero. Then we have proved the first statement of the following proposition.

Proposition 3.12 *The estimator* $\bar{y}_{\mathrm{rss}}^* = \bar{\bar{y}}_{\mathrm{rss}}\left(\frac{a\bar{x}_{\mathrm{rss}}+b}{a\bar{x}_{s^*}+b}\right)^\alpha\left(\frac{a\bar{x}_{\mathrm{rss}}+b}{a\bar{x}_{s^*}+b}\right)^\beta$ *is asymptotically unbiased in terms of* n *and its variance is given by*

$$V(\bar{\bar{y}}_{\mathrm{rss}}^*) = \frac{\sigma_Y^2}{n} + \gamma\mu_Y^2\left(((\alpha+\beta)\phi)^2 c_x^2 + 2(\alpha+\beta)\phi K_{xy}c_x^2 + \frac{\Psi_{XY}}{\mu_x\mu_Y}\right)$$

$$+ \lambda\mu_{Y_2}^2\left(\frac{\sigma_{Y_2}^2}{\mu_{Y_2}^2} + \frac{\Psi_{Y_2}}{\mu_{Y_2}^2} + \alpha\phi\left(\alpha\phi\left(\frac{\sigma_x^2}{\mu_x^2} + \Psi_{x_2}\right)\right) + 2(K_{x_2Y}c_{x_2}^2)\right.$$

$$\left. + \frac{\Psi_{X_2Y}}{\mu_x\mu_Y}(1 + \Psi_{x_2}) + \frac{\sigma_{x_2Y}^2}{\mu_x\mu_Y}\right)$$

if $/\phi Z/ < 1, Z = \varepsilon_{\mathrm{rss}}, \theta_{\mathrm{rss}}, \vartheta, \omega_{\mathrm{rss}}$.

Proof An expansion in Taylor Series of $(\bar{\bar{y}}_{\mathrm{rss}}^* - \mu_Y)^2$ may be worked out. It is neglecting the terms of order $t > 2$,

$$(\bar{\bar{y}}_{\mathrm{rss}}^* - \mu_Y)^2 = \mu_Y^2(\tau_1 + \tau_2 + \tau_3 + \tau_4)$$

where

$$\tau_1 = \varepsilon_{rss}^2 + (\alpha^2\theta_{rss}^2 + \beta^2\omega_{rss}^2 + 2\alpha\beta\varepsilon_{rss}\omega_{rss})\phi^2$$
$$\tau_2 = \varepsilon_{rss}^2 + (\alpha+\beta)^2\vartheta^2\phi^2$$
$$\tau_3 = 2\phi(\alpha\varepsilon_{rss}\theta_{rss} + \beta\varepsilon_{rss}\omega_{rss})$$
$$\tau_4 = -2(\alpha+\beta)(\phi\vartheta\varepsilon_{rss} + \phi^2(\alpha\vartheta\varepsilon_{rss} + \beta\vartheta\omega_{rss}))$$

Calculating the expected value and grouping we have that

$$E(\bar{y}_{rss}^* - \mu_Y)^2 = \frac{\sigma_Y^2}{n} + \gamma\mu_Y^2\left(((\alpha+\beta)\phi)^2 c_x^2 + 2(\alpha+\beta)\phi K_{xy}c_x^2 + \frac{\Psi_{XY}}{\mu_x\mu_Y}\right)$$
$$+ \lambda\mu_{Y_2}^2\left(\frac{\sigma_{Y_2}^2}{\mu_{Y_2}^2} + \frac{\Psi_{Y_2}}{\mu_{Y_2}^2} + \alpha\phi\left(\alpha\phi\left(\frac{\sigma_x^2}{\mu_x^2} + \Psi_{x_2}\right)\right) + 2(K_{x_2Y}c_{x_2}^2)$$
$$+ \frac{\Psi_{X_2Y}}{\mu_x\mu_Y}(1+\Psi_{x_2}) + \frac{\sigma_{x_2Y}^2}{\mu_x\mu_Y}\right) \qquad \square$$

Remark 3.13 The gain in accuracy due to the use of $\bar{y}_{rss}^*$ in terms of the variance is
$$G_{rss} = \frac{\sigma_{x_2y} + \gamma\mu_y^2\Psi_{xy} + 2\Psi_{xy}(1+\Psi_2) + \lambda\Psi_{x_2}\mu_y^2}{\mu_x\mu_y} \qquad \square$$

Hence, as $V(\bar{y}_{rss}^*) = V(\bar{y}^*) + G$ the proposed method is more precise if $G < 0$.

This result allows deducing the RSS counterparts of different double sampling estimators of the mean. For example

$(\alpha, \beta, a, b) = (-1, 0, 1, 0) \rightarrow$ Khare - Srivastava - Tabasum - Khan estimator 1
$(\alpha, \beta, a, b) = (0, -1, 1, 0) \rightarrow$ Khare - Srivastava - Tabasum - Khan estimator 2
$(\alpha, \beta, a, b) = (-1, -1, 1, 0) \rightarrow$ Singh - Kumar ratio estimator
$(\alpha, \beta, a, b) = (-1, 0, 1, 0) \rightarrow$ Singh - Kumar product estimator

See Khare and Srivastava (1993), Singh, H. P and Kumar, S (2008a, b, 2009).

References

Agrawal, M. C., Sthapit, A. B. (1997). Hierarchic predictive ratio-based and product-based estimators and their efficiency. *Journal of Applied Statistics*, 24, 97–104.

Bouza, C. N., & Prabhu-Ajgaonkar, S. G. (1993). Estimation of the difference of population means when observations are missing. *Biometrical Journal, 35*, 245–252.

Bouza, C. N. (1983). Estimation of the difference of population means with missing observations. *Biometrical Journal, 25*, 123–128.

Bouza, C. N. (2001). Random set sampling with non-responses. *Revista de Matemática e Estatística, 19*, 297–308.

Bouza, C. N. (2002). Ranked set sub sampling the nonresponse strata for estimating the difference of means. *Biometrical Journal, 44*, 903–915.

Bouza, C. N. (2008). Estimation of the population mean with missing observations using product type estimators. *Revista Investigación Operacional, 29*, 207–223.

Bouza, C. N. (1981a). Bias and NR rate reduction using a RR model among the NR. Survey Statistician, 1–5.

Bouza, C. N. (1981b). Sobre el problema de la fracciòn de muestreo para el caso de las no respuestas. *Trabajos de Estadística, 21*, 18–24.

Bouza, C. N. (2011). Handling with missing observations in simple random sampling and rankedset sampling. *International Encyclopedia of Statistical Science part 8*, 621–622.

Cochran, W. G. (1977). *Sampling techniques*. New York: Wiley.

David, I. P., & Sukhatme, B. V. (1974). On the bias and mean square error of the ratio estimator. *Journal of the American Statistical Association, 69*, 464.

Hansen, M. H., & Hurwitz, W. N. (1946). The problem of non responses in sample surveys. *Journal of the American Statistical Association, 41*, 517–529.

Khare, B. B., & Srivastava, S. (1993). Estimation of population mean using auxiliary character in presence of non-response. *National Academy of Sciences, India, 16*, 111–114.

Muttlak, H. A. (1996). Median ranked set sampling. *Journal of Applied Statistical Science, 6*, 91–98.

Pi-ehr, L. (1971). Estimation procedures for the difference of means with missing observations. *Journal of the American Statistical Association*, 41, 517–553.

Samawi, H., Abu-Dayyeh, W., & Ahmed, S. (1996). Extreme ranked set sampling. *Biometrical Journal, 30*, 577–586.

Karl-erik, S., Särndal, K-E., & Lundström, S. (2005). *Estimation in surveys with nonresponse*. Chichester: Wiley.

Singh, S. (2003). *Advanced sampling theory with applications*, kluwer. Dordrecht, Amsterdam: Academic publishers.

Singh, H. P., Kumar, S. (2008a). Estimation of mean in presence on non response using two phase sampling scheme. *Statistical Papers*. doi 10.1007/s00362-008-01040-5.

Singh, H. P., & Kumar, S. (2008b). A regression approach to the estimation of finite population mean in presence on non response. *Australian and New Zealand Journal of Statistics, 50*, 395–408.

Singh, H. P., & Kumar, S. (2009). A general procedure of estimating the population mean in the presence under double sampling using auxiliary information. *Statistics and Operations Research Transactions, 33*, 71–84.

Srinath, K. P. (1971). Multi-phase sampling in non-response problems. *Journal of the American Statistical Association, 66*, 583–589.

Chapter 4
Imputation of the Missing Data

Abstract We may consider the existence of missing observations as unimportant, considering that the risk of misunderstanding is negligible. The surveyor assumes some model that allows adequately explaining the variable of interest. In such cases, we are able to predict the unknown values and to plug them into some estimator. Generally, the models used for imputing in sampling are not complicated and rely on simple ideas. Imputation in simple random sampling has been developed for decades; the literature is increased yearly. Ranked Set Sampling (RSS) alternatives are presented in this chapter. The efficiency of this approach is supported for the different models. On some occasions the preference of RSS is doubtful and needs numerical comparisons.

Keywords Imputation procedures · Ignorable case · Missing at random · Expected variance · SRS · RSS · Efficiency

> *Let us act on what we have, since we have not what we wish.*
> Cardinal Newman

4.1 Introduction

The use of imputation techniques for dealing with missing information is a theme of actuality. See for example, Chang-Huang (2000a, b, 2001), Rueda and González (2004), Rueda et al. (2006), Tsukerman (2004), Young-Jae (2005), Liu et al. (2006), Zou et al. (2002).

Rubin (1976), classified missing data mechanisms into three types.

1. Missing completely at random (MCAR). This mechanism is characterized by a distribution such that the probability that a value is missing is independent of values (observed or missing) in the dataset. Hence the observed value of Y is a

C. N. Bouza-Herrera, *Handling Missing Data in Ranked Set Sampling*, 59
SpringerBriefs in Statistics, DOI: 10.1007/978-3-642-39899-5_4,

random result from the set of observed and unobserved values. That is any sampled unit from the population is representative and the subsample interviewed is a representative subsample of the selected sample.

2. Missing at random (MAR). The distribution that characterizes it is such that if Y is missing in a unit and may depend on some observed values in the dataset but is independent of any missing data. Then the subsample interviewed is not a representative subsample of those selected. An appropriate analysis needs to be used to address the bias.

3. Not missing at random (NMAR). If missing data cannot be considered that are generated neither by MCAR nor by MAR the probability that Y be missing may be generated by a dependence on missing data. A NMAR mechanism is present when the missing values are systematically different from observed values, even after conditioning on observed values. Any statistical procedure is expected to behave inaccurately if the missing data mechanism is NMAR.

Weighting adjustment is often used to compensate for unit non-response. Imputation is usually used to compensate for item non-response. Imputation is widely used in sample surveys to assign values for item non-responses. If the imputed values are treated as if they were observed, then the estimates of the variances of the estimator will be increased. If a bias is present, the square of it is present in the sampling error. When only the responses are used the estimates will generally be underestimations. Methods for imputing missing data in survey sampling under various cases of item non-response are of importance.

When the non-response mechanism can be evaluated as MCAR or MAR the missing data may be classified as ignorable. The term ignorable is used for establishing that it is not necessary specifying it explicitly. That is, the missing data mechanism can be ignored. In any case, the statistical analysis should take the missing data for diminishing the bias of the estimators. Hence, though the missing data mechanism that is ignorable, the existence of missing data must be taken into account. Procedures using of the responses and ignoring the missing observations is commonly identified as "amputation" as a counterpart of "imputation".

If MCAR is the NR mechanism we may consider the so-called complete-case analysis. It discards the need of considering the subjects missing. It is the simplest procedure for handling missing data. It is usually done automatically by most software packages when missing data are present. If the mechanism is not MCAR it produces biased estimates.

Different imputation procedures are commonly used in practice.

The procedure called mean substitution is typically implemented by replacing a missing value with the average of the observed values, and analyzing the dataset as if it were complete. It does not take into account uncertainty in the true but unknown value. It is used both for MCA and MR responses mechanisms.

Single imputation is a general method of replacing missing values with values derived ad hoc. The imputed values have the same distribution as the non-missing data. For each sampled unit having any missing data, a substitution model uses some available non-missing data of it to form a predictor. Once each missing value that imputed the estimator uses the completed dataset. This procedure has the advantage of replacing missing data with values whose distributions are like the non-missing ones. For an imputation procedure to be valid, it must take into account the fact that imputed values are only a guess and not the value that would have been observed and not the missing values. It is typically used in the presence of a MAR mechanism.

In the sequel, we present results on imputation for RSS which extend recent results on imputing under srswr.

4.2 Ignoring the Non-responses in the Estimation of the Mean

Surveyors have ignored the non-responses since the beginnings of surveying using random samples. See Chen et al. (2004), Toutenburg et al. (2008), (Bai and Chen 2003).

Consider $\mu_z = \frac{\sum_{i=1}^{N} z_i}{N,}$, and $\sigma_z^2, z = X, Y$ to be the population mean and variance and ρ as the correlation coefficient between X and Y. Y is the variable of interest, which presumably exhibits some missing values pattern, X is a known variable. X may be known for all the units in the population or, at least, for all the units in the sample.

Let k be the number of responding units, out of the sampled n units selected using simple random sampling method with replacement (SRSWR) from a population of size N. The respondents sample is given by:

$$\bar{y}_s = \frac{1}{k} \sum_{i=1}^{k} y_i,$$

with variance $V(\bar{y}_s) = \frac{\sigma_y^2}{k}$. A MCAR mechanism is assumed and the probability P obtaining a response at a visit is a constant and $E(\bar{y}_k) = \mu_y$.

Under this mechanism we can use the mean substitution method. Define

$$y_i^* = \begin{cases} y_i & \text{if } i \text{ responds} \\ \bar{y}_s & \text{if } i \text{ does not respond} \end{cases}$$

and use the sample mean of the defined variables

$$\bar{y}_m^* = \frac{\sum_{i=1}^{n} y_i^*}{n}$$

As $E(\bar{y}_s) = \mu_y$ we have that $E(\bar{y}_m^*) = \mu_y$ and

$$V(\bar{y}_m^*) = \frac{k\sigma_y^2 + (n-k)\frac{\sigma_y^2}{n}}{n^2} = \frac{n + k(n-1)}{n^3}\sigma_y^2$$

Note that when $k = n$ it attains the srswr value $\frac{\sigma_y^2}{n}$.

The ratio method suggests the naïve point estimator of the population mean

$$\bar{y}_k = \frac{\bar{y}_s}{\bar{x}_s}\bar{x},$$

where $\bar{x}_s = \frac{1}{k}\sum_{i=1}^{k} x_i$. is the sample mean of X under the mean method of ignorability of the missing values and $\bar{x} = \frac{\sum_{i=1}^{n} x_i}{n}$ is the sample mean based on n units with variance $V(\bar{x}) = \frac{\sigma_x^2}{n}$.

As we have a random sample of size k, from standard results of the theory of ratio estimation, the bias and mean square error (MSE) of $\bar{y}_k$ are

$$B(\bar{y}_k) \cong \left(\frac{1}{k} - \frac{1}{n}\right)\left(C_x^2 - \rho C_y C_x\right)\mu_y$$

$$\text{MSE}(\bar{y}_k) \cong \frac{\sigma_y^2}{k} + \left(\frac{1}{k} - \frac{1}{n}\right)\left(R^2\sigma_X^2 - 2R\sigma_{XY}\right)$$

where $C_Z = \frac{\sigma_Z}{\mu_Z}$, $Z = X, Y$, $R = \frac{\mu_y}{\mu_x}$, $\rho = \frac{\sigma_{XY}}{\sigma_X\sigma_Y}$, and σ_{xy} is the covariance between X and Y. Note that if $k \cong n$ the bias is close to zero.

We have that, $\bar{y}_k$ is more efficient than $\bar{y}_s$ if $\frac{C_x}{C_y} < 2\rho$ for $R > 0$ and $\frac{C_x}{C_y} > 2\rho$ for $R < 0$.

4.3 Ratio Imputation Procedures

4.3.1 SRWR Designs

Kadilar and Cingi (2008) considered the case of missing data in estimating the population suggesting the following estimators of the population mean of the study variable Y:

$$\bar{y}_{KC1} = \frac{\bar{y}_s + b(\mu_x - \bar{x})}{\bar{x}}\mu_x, \quad \bar{y}_{KC2} = \frac{\bar{y}_s + b(\mu_x - \bar{x}_s)}{\bar{x}_s}\mu_x, \quad \bar{y}_{KC3} = \frac{\bar{y}_s + b(\bar{x} - \bar{x}_s)}{\bar{x}_s}\bar{x}$$

where $b = \frac{s_{xy}}{s_x^2}$ is the regression coefficient, s_{xy} is the sample covariance between X and Y, and s_x^2 is the sample variance of X. Their biases are

$$B(\bar{y}_{KC1}) \cong \frac{C_x^2\mu_y}{n}, \quad B(\bar{y}_{KC2}) \cong \frac{C_x^2\mu_y}{k}, \quad B(\bar{y}_{KC3}) \cong \left(\frac{1}{k} - \frac{1}{n}\right)\rho C_x C_y\mu_y,$$

respectively. The mean square errors of these estimators are

$$\text{MSE}(\bar{y}_{\text{KC1}}) \cong \frac{\sigma_y^2}{k} + \frac{(R^2 - B^2)\sigma_x^2}{n}$$

$$\text{MSE}(\bar{y}_{\text{KC2}}) \cong \frac{1}{k}(\sigma_y^2 - B\sigma_{xy} + R^2\sigma_x^2)$$

$$\text{MSE}(\bar{y}_{\text{KC3}}) \cong \frac{\sigma_y^2}{k} + \left(\frac{1}{k} - \frac{1}{n}\right)(R^2 - B^2)\sigma_x^2$$

where $B = \frac{\sigma_{xy}}{\sigma_x^2} = \frac{\rho\sigma_y}{\sigma_x}$.

Singh and Horn (2000) suggested a ratio estimator of the population mean in the form

$$\bar{y}_{\text{SH}} = \alpha\bar{y}_s + (1 - \alpha)\frac{\bar{y}_s\bar{x}}{\bar{x}_s}$$

the value of which makes the MSE minimum is $\alpha_0 = 1 - \rho\frac{C_y}{C_x}$. The bias and MSE of $\bar{y}_{\text{SH}}$ respectively are

$$B(\bar{y}_{\text{SH}}) \cong (1 - \alpha)\left(\frac{1}{k} - \frac{1}{n}\right)(C_x^2 - \rho C_y C_x)\mu_y,$$

and

$$\text{MSE}_{\min}(\bar{y}_{\text{SH}}) \cong \text{MSE}(\bar{y}_k) - \left(\frac{1}{k} - \frac{1}{n}\right)\left(1 - \rho\frac{C_y}{C_x}\right)\mu_y C_x^2$$

Singh and Deo (2003) considered the estimator

$$\bar{y}_{\text{SD}} = \bar{y}_s\left(\frac{\bar{x}}{\bar{x}_s}\right)^\lambda,$$

using $\lambda = \rho\frac{C_y}{C_x}$. The bias and MSE of $\bar{y}_{\text{SD}}$, respectively are

$$B(\bar{y}_{\text{SD}}) \cong \left(\frac{1}{k} - \frac{1}{n}\right)\left(\frac{\lambda(\lambda - 1)}{2}C_x^2 - \lambda\rho C_y C_x\right)\mu_y,$$

and

$$\text{MSE}_{\min}(\bar{y}_{\text{SD}}) \cong \text{MSE}(\bar{y}_k) - \left(\frac{1}{k} - \frac{1}{n}\right)(B - R)^2\sigma_x^2$$

Al-Omari and Jaber (2008), Al-Omari et al. (2008), Al-Omari et al. (2009) considered ratio-type estimators using the knowledge of the first or the third quartiles of the auxiliary variable X. The suggested estimators had the structure

$$\bar{y}_{1q_h} = \bar{y}_s \left(\frac{\mu_x + q_h}{\bar{x} + q_h} \right)$$

where q_1 and q_3 are the first and third quartiles of the auxiliary variable X. For simplicity we denote these classes of estimators by the order of the quartile $h = 1, 3$. Using Taylor Series approximation, the estimators can be written as

$$\bar{y}_{1q_h} \cong \bar{y}_s - T_h(\bar{x} - \mu_x) + T_h G_h(\bar{x} - \mu_x)^2 - G_h(\bar{x} - \mu_x)(\bar{y} - \mu_y)$$

where $T_h = \frac{\mu_y}{\mu_x + q_h}, G_h = \frac{1}{\mu_x + q_h}, h = 1, 3$. For the first degree of approximation the estimator is given by $\bar{y}_{1q_h} \cong \bar{y}_s - T_h(\bar{x} - \mu_x)$. Calculating its expectation is derived that

$$E(\bar{y}_{1q_h}) \cong E(\bar{y}_s) - T_h(\bar{x} - \mu_x) = \mu_y$$

Then $B(\bar{y}_{1q_h}) \cong 0$. Since the estimator is approximately unbiased the variance and MSE are approximately equal. As $B = \frac{\sigma_{xy}}{\sigma_x^2} = \frac{\rho \sigma_y}{\sigma_x}$, and $\text{Cov}(\bar{x}, \bar{y}_s) = \frac{\rho \sigma_x \sigma_y}{n}$ we have that

$$\text{MSE}(\bar{y}_{1q_h}) \cong V(\bar{y}_s) + T_h^2 V(\bar{x}) - 2T_h \text{Cov}(\bar{x}, \bar{y}_s) = \frac{\sigma_y^2}{k} + \frac{T_h \sigma_x^2 (T_h - 2B)}{n}$$

The second suggested class of estimators is

$$\bar{y}_{2q_h} = \bar{y} \left(\frac{\mu_x + q_h}{\bar{x}_s + q_h} \right)$$

where $h = 1, 3$. Using Taylor series approximation this estimator can be expressed by

$$\bar{y}_{2q_h} \cong \bar{y} - T_h(\bar{x}_s - \mu_x) + T_h G_h(\bar{x}_s - \mu_x)^2 - G_h(\bar{x}_s - \mu_x)(\bar{y} - \mu_y)$$

and the first degree of approximation the estimator is given by $\bar{y}_{2q_h} \cong \bar{y}_s - T_h(\bar{x}_s - \mu_x)$.

The bias of $\bar{y}_{2q_h}$ is $B(\bar{y}_{2q_h}) \cong 0$, and

$$\text{MSE}(\bar{y}_{2q_h}) \cong V(\bar{y}_s) + T_h^2 V(\bar{x}) - 2T_h \text{Cov}(\bar{x}, \bar{y}_s) = \frac{\sigma_y^2}{n} + \frac{T_h^2 \sigma_x^2 (T_h - 2B)}{k} - \frac{2T_h B \sigma_x^2}{n}$$

The third class of Bouza and Al-Omari (2013) estimators is

$$\bar{y}_{3q_h} = \bar{y}_s \left(\frac{\mu_x + q_h}{\bar{x}_s + q_h} \right)$$

where $h = 1, 3$. Using again Taylor Series approximation for the first degree this estimator is derived

$$\bar{y}_{3q_h} \cong \bar{y}_s - T_h(\bar{x}_s - \mu_x) + T_h G_h(\bar{x}_s - \mu_x)^2 - G_h(\bar{x}_s - \mu_x)(\bar{y}_s - \mu_y),$$

Its first degree of approximation is $\bar{y}_{3q_h} \cong \bar{y}_s - T_h(\bar{x}_s - \mu_x)$. The bias of this class of estimators has a similar behavior and $B(\bar{y}_{23}) \cong 0$ the MSE is:

$$\mathrm{MSE}\left(\bar{y}_{3q_h}\right) \cong V(\bar{y}_s) + T_h^2 V(\bar{x}_s) - 2T_h \mathrm{Cov}(\bar{x}_s, \bar{y}_s) = \frac{\sigma_y^2 + T_h^2 \sigma_x^2 - 2T_h B \sigma_x^2}{k}$$

The efficiency of the classes of estimators under SRSWR provides an insight for selecting to use one of them under certain circumstances.

The efficiency of the estimators $\bar{y}_{tq_h}, t = 1, 2, 3, h = 1, 2$ is established comparing the corresponding MSE's.

$\bar{y}_{1q_h}$ and $\bar{y}_{3q_h}$ are more efficient than $\bar{y}_s$ if $T_h < 2B$ and $\bar{y}_{2q_h}$ is more efficient than $\bar{y}_s$ if $\left(\frac{1}{k} - \frac{1}{n}\right)\sigma_y^2 + \frac{\sigma_x^2 T_h (T_h - 2B)}{k} < 0$. The condition

$$\left(\frac{1}{n}\right) T_h (T_h - 2B) - \left(\frac{1}{k} - \frac{1}{n}\right)(R - 2B) < 0$$

supports that $\bar{y}_{1q_h}$, is more efficient than $\bar{y}_k$. The condition

$$2T_h \sigma_x^2 \left(\frac{T_h}{k} - \frac{2B}{n}\right) + \left(\frac{1}{k} - \frac{1}{n}\right)(2RB\sigma_x^2 - R^2\sigma_x^2 - \sigma_y^2) < 0$$

provides the same conclusion for $\bar{y}_{2q_h}$ and $\bar{y}_{3q_h}$ is more efficient when

$$\left(\frac{1}{k}\right) T_h (T_h - 2B) - \left(\frac{1}{k} - \frac{1}{n}\right) R(R - 2B) < 0$$

Therefore, the knowledge of certain parameters allows establishing which criteria provides more efficiency estimation when compared with $\bar{y}_k$.

The efficiency of these classes with respect to Kadilar and Cingi (2008) estimators are fixed similarly.

We have that the estimators of type $\bar{y}_{1q_h}$ are more efficient than Kadilar and Cingi (2008) estimators under the following conditions:

- $\bar{y}_{1q_h}$ is better than $\bar{y}_{KC1}$ if $T_h^2 + B^2 - R^2 - 2T_h B < 0$
- $\bar{y}_{1q_h}$ is better than $\bar{y}_{KC2}$ if $\left(\frac{1}{n}\right)\left(T_h^2 - 2T_h B\right) - \left(\frac{1}{k}\right)(B^2 - R^2) < 0$
- $\bar{y}_{1q_h}$ is better than $\bar{y}_{KC3}$ if $\left(\frac{1}{n}\right)\left(T_h^2 - 2T_h B\right) - \left(\frac{1}{k} - \frac{1}{n}\right)(B^2 - R^2) < 0$

For estimators of type $\bar{y}_{2q_h}$ the conditions of efficiency are

- $\bar{y}_{2q_h}$ is better than $\bar{y}_{KC1}$ if $\frac{T_h^2 \sigma_x^2 - \sigma_y^2}{k} + \frac{\sigma_y^2 - 2T_h B \sigma_x^2 - \sigma_x^2 (R^2 - B^2)}{n} < 0$
- $\bar{y}_{2q_h}$ is better than $\bar{y}_{KC2}$ if $\frac{(T_h^2 + B^2 - R^2)\sigma_x^2 - \sigma_y^2}{k} + \frac{\sigma_y^2 - 2T_h B \sigma_x^2}{n} < 0$
- $\bar{y}_{2q_h}$ is better than $\bar{y}_{KC3}$ if

$$\frac{T_h^2 \sigma_x^2 - \sigma_y^2}{k} + \frac{\sigma_y^2 - 2T_h B \sigma_x^2}{n} + \left(\frac{1}{k} - \frac{1}{n}\right)\left[(R + B)^2 \sigma_x^2 - 2(R + B)\sigma_{xy}\right] < 0$$

The conditions for preferring the estimators of type $\bar{y}_{3q_h}$ are:

- $\bar{y}_{3q_h}$ is better than $\bar{y}_{KC1}$ if $\left(\frac{1}{k}\right)\left(T_h^2 - 2T_h B\right) - \left(\frac{1}{n}\right)\left(R^2 - B^2\right) < 0$
- $\bar{y}_{3q_h}$ is better than $\bar{y}_{KC2}$ if $T_h^2 - 2T_h B - R^2 + B^2 < 0$
- $\bar{y}_{3q_h}$ is better than $\bar{y}_{KC3}$ if $\frac{T_h^2 - 2T_h B}{k} - \left(\frac{1}{k} - \frac{1}{n}\right)\left[R^2 - B^2\right] < 0$

The efficiency with respect to Singh and Horn (2000) and Singh and Deo (2003) estimators is derived using the fact that the MSE the estimators proposed can be rewritten as

$$\text{MSE}_{\min}(\bar{y}_{\text{SH}}) = \text{MSE}_{\min}(\bar{y}_{\text{SD}}) \cong \frac{\sigma_y^2}{k} - \left(\frac{1}{k} - \frac{1}{n}\right) B^2 \sigma_x^2$$

The efficiency of the quartiles based classes of ratio-type estimators developed is characterized as follows:

- $\bar{y}_{1q_h}$ is more efficient than $\bar{y}_{\text{SD}}$ and $\bar{y}_{\text{SH}}$ if $\left(\frac{1}{n}\right)\left(T_h^2 - 2T_h B\right) - \left(\frac{1}{k} - \frac{1}{n}\right) B^2 < 0$
- $\bar{y}_{2q_h}$ is more efficient than $\bar{y}_{\text{SD}}$ and $\bar{y}_{\text{SH}}$ if
-

$$\frac{T_h^2 \sigma_x^2 - \sigma_y^2}{k} + \frac{\sigma_y^2 - 2T_h B \sigma_x^2}{n} + \left(\frac{1}{k} - \frac{1}{n}\right)\left(\frac{1}{k} - \frac{1}{n}\right) B^2 \sigma_x^2 < 0$$

- $\bar{y}_{3q_h}$ is more efficient than $\bar{y}_{\text{SD}}$ and $\bar{y}_{\text{SH}}$ if $\frac{T_h^2 - 2T_h B}{k} + \left(\frac{1}{k} - \frac{1}{n}\right) B^2 < 0$

Another class was considered by Bouza and Al-Omari (2011c) exploiting the fact that the correlation coefficient between X and Y, ρ is known. They are given by:

$$\bar{y}_{1\rho} = \bar{y}_s \left(\frac{\mu_x + \rho}{\bar{x} + \rho}\right), \ \bar{y}_{2\rho} = \bar{y}\left(\frac{\mu_x + \rho}{\bar{x}_s + \rho}\right), \ \bar{y}_{3\rho} = \bar{y}_s \left(\frac{\mu_x + \rho}{\bar{x}_s + \rho}\right)$$

Their Taylor Series approximations are

$$\bar{y}_{1\rho} \cong \bar{y}_s - D(\bar{x} - \mu_x) + DL(\bar{x} - \mu_x)^2 - L(\bar{x} - \mu_x)(\bar{y} - \mu_y)$$
$$\bar{y}_{2\rho} \cong \bar{y} - D(\bar{x}_s - \mu_x) + DL(\bar{x}_s - \mu_x)^2 - L(\bar{x}_s - \mu_x)(\bar{y} - \mu_y)$$
$$\bar{y}_{3\rho} \cong \bar{y}_s - D(\bar{x}_s - \mu_x) + DL(\bar{x}_s - \mu_x)^2 - L(\bar{x}_s - \mu_x)(\bar{y} - \mu_y)$$

where $D = \frac{\mu_y}{\mu_x + \rho}, L = \frac{1}{\mu_x + \rho}$, for the first degree of approximation, the estimator is given by

$$\bar{y}_{1\rho} \cong \bar{y}_s - D(\bar{x} - \mu_x), \bar{y}_{2\rho} \cong \bar{y} - D(\bar{x}_s - \mu_x) \text{ and } \bar{y}_{3\rho} \cong \bar{y}_s - D(\bar{x}_s - \mu_x).$$ They are approximately unbiased as $D(E(\bar{x}) - \mu_x) = D(E(\bar{x}_s) - \mu_x) = 0$. Their MSE's are

$$\text{MSE}(\bar{y}_{1\rho}) \cong \frac{\sigma_Y^2}{k} + \frac{1}{n}\left(D\sigma_X^2(D-2B)\right), \; B = \frac{\sigma_{XY}}{\sigma_X^2} = \frac{\rho\sigma_Y}{\sigma_X}$$

$$\text{MSE}(\bar{y}_{2\rho}) \cong \frac{\sigma_Y^2}{n} + \frac{D^2\sigma_X^2}{k} - \frac{2DB\sigma_X^2}{n}$$

$$\text{MSE}(\bar{y}_{3\rho}) \cong \frac{1}{k}\left(\sigma_Y^2 + D^2\sigma_X^2 - 2DB\sigma_X^2\right)$$

Noting that the estimators are approximately unbiased, it is clear that the variance and MSE are equal approximately.

The suggested estimators are easily evaluated considering that

- $\bar{y}_{1\rho}$ and $\bar{y}_{3\rho}$ are more efficient than $\bar{y}_s$ if $D < 2B$.
- $\bar{y}_{2\rho}$ is more efficient than $\bar{y}_s$ if $\left(\frac{1}{k} - \frac{1}{n}\right)\sigma_Y^2 + \frac{1}{k}\left(\sigma_X^2 D(D-2B)\right) < 0$.
- $\bar{y}_{1\rho}$ is more efficient than $\bar{y}_k$ if $\frac{1}{n}D(D-2B) - \left(\frac{1}{k} - \frac{1}{n}\right)(R-2B) < 0$.
- $\bar{y}_{2\rho}$ is more efficient than $\bar{y}_k$ if $\left(\frac{1}{k} - \frac{1}{n}\right)\left(2RB\sigma_X^2 - R^2\sigma_X^2 - \sigma_Y^2\right) + \left(\frac{D}{k} - \frac{2B}{n}\right)$ $2D\sigma_X^2 < 0$.
- $\bar{y}_{3\rho}$ is more efficient than $\bar{y}_k$ if $\frac{1}{k}D(D-2B) - \left(\frac{1}{k} - \frac{1}{n}\right)R(R-2B) < 0$.

A comparison with the estimators, proposed by Kadilar and Cingi (2008), should be based on considering that

- $\bar{y}_{1\rho}$ is more efficient than $\bar{y}_{\text{KC1}}$ if $D^2 + B^2 - R^2 - 2DB < 0$.
- $\bar{y}_{1\rho}$ is more efficient than $\bar{y}_{\text{KC2}}$ if $\frac{1}{n}\left(D^2 - 2DB\right) + \frac{1}{k}\left(B^2 - R^2\right) < 0$.
- $\bar{y}_{1\rho}$ is more efficient than $\bar{y}_{\text{KC3}}$ if $\frac{1}{n}\left(D^2 - 2DB\right) - \left(\frac{1}{k} - \frac{1}{n}\right)\left(B^2 - R^2\right) < 0$.

An analysis of $\bar{y}_{2\rho}$ leads to establish as efficiency conditions

- It is more efficient than $\bar{y}_{\text{KC1}}$ if
-

$$\frac{1}{k}\left[D^2\sigma_X^2 - \sigma_Y^2\right] + \frac{1}{n}\left[\sigma_Y^2 - 2DB\sigma_X^2 - \sigma_X^2\left(R^2 - B^2\right)\right] < 0.$$

- It is more efficient than $\bar{y}_{\text{KC2}}$ if
-

$$\frac{1}{k}\left[(D^2 + B^2 - R^2)\sigma_X^2 - \sigma_Y^2\right] + \frac{1}{n}\left[\sigma_Y^2 - 2DB\sigma_X^2\right] < 0.$$

- It is more efficient than $\bar{y}_{\text{KC3}}$ if

$$\frac{1}{k}\left[D^2\sigma_X^2 - \sigma_Y^2\right] + \frac{1}{n}\left[\sigma_Y^2 - 2DB\sigma_X^2\right] + \left(\frac{1}{k} - \frac{1}{n}\right)\left[(R+B)^2\sigma_X^2 - 2(R+B)\sigma_{XY}\right] < 0.$$

A similar analysis of $\bar{y}_{3\rho}$ fixes that

- $\bar{y}_{3\rho}$ is more efficient than $\bar{y}_{KC1}$ if $\frac{1}{k}\left(D^2 - 2DB\right) - \frac{1}{n}\left(R^2 - B^2\right) < 0$.
- $\bar{y}_{3\rho}$ is more efficient than $\bar{y}_{KC2}$ if $\left(D - B\right)^2 - R^2 < 0$.
- $\bar{y}_{3\rho}$ is more efficient than $\bar{y}_{KC3}$ if $\frac{1}{k}\left(D^2 - 2DB\right) - \left(\frac{1}{k} - \frac{1}{n}\right)\left(R^2 - B^2\right) < 0$.

A comparison of the MSE of the estimators of Singh and Horn (2000) and Singh and Deo (2003) yields that

- $\bar{y}_{1\rho}$ is more efficient than $\bar{y}_{SD}$ and $\bar{y}_{SH}$ if $\frac{1}{n}\left(D^2 - 2DB\right) + \left(\frac{1}{k} - \frac{1}{n}\right)B^2 < 0$.
- $\bar{y}_{2\rho}$ is more efficient than $\bar{y}_{SD}$ and $\bar{y}_{SH}$ because

$$\frac{1}{k}\left(D^2\sigma_X^2 - \sigma_Y^2\right) + \frac{1}{n}\left(\sigma_Y^2 - 2DB\sigma_X^2\right) + \left(\frac{1}{k} - \frac{1}{n}\right)B^2\sigma_X^2 < 0.$$

- $\bar{y}_{3\rho}$ is more efficient than $\bar{y}_{SD}$ and $\bar{y}_{SH}$ if $\frac{1}{k}\left(D^2 - 2DB\right) + \left(\frac{1}{k} - \frac{1}{n}\right)B^2 < 0$.

4.3.2 The RSS Design

The case of SRSWR can be extended to RSS using the relationships between the sample mean and the average of the os's. The existence of missing observations establishes that for each order statistic there are only $r(j)$ responses, $1 \le r(j) \le r$. Hence $k = \sum_{j=1}^{m} r(j)$.

The existence of missing observations establishes that, for each os, there are only $r(j)$ responses, $1 \le r(j) \le r$. Following the line of considering only the elements that respond can use

$$\bar{z}'_{(rss)} = \frac{1}{m}\sum_{j=1}^{m}\frac{\sum_{k}^{r(j)} z_{(j:j)k}}{r(j)}$$

it is an unbiased estimator of the population mean of $Z = X, Y$ because

$$E\left(\bar{z}'_{(rss)}\right) = \frac{1}{m}\sum_{j=1}^{m}\frac{\sum_{k}^{r(j)}\mu_{Z(j)}}{r(j)} = \frac{1}{m}\sum_{j=1}^{m}\mu_{Z(j)}$$

due to the property of the os, see Takahasi and Wakimoto (1968). As the samples are independent and they were selected using srswr the variance is given by

$$V\left(\bar{z}'_{(rss)}\right) = \frac{1}{m^2}\sum_{j=1}^{m}\frac{\sum_{k}^{r(j)}\sigma_{z(j)}^2}{r(j)^2} = \frac{\sigma_z^2}{m^2}\sum_{j=1}^{m}r(j)^{-1} - \frac{1}{m^2}\sum_{j=1}^{m}D_{z(j)}^2 r(j)^{-1}$$

using the fact that the variance of an os is $\sigma_{Z(j)}^2 = \sigma_Z^2 - D_{Z(j)}^2$, $D_{z(j)} = \mu_{z(j)} - \mu_z$.

Take $Z = X$, then the counterpart of $\bar{y}_k$ is $\bar{y}_{(rss)}$. Hence the use of RSS is measured by

$$G(\bar{y}_k, \bar{y}'_{(rss)}) = V(\bar{y}_k) - V\left(\bar{y}'_{(rss)}\right) = \sigma_Y^2\left(\frac{1}{k} - \frac{1}{m^2}\sum_{j=1}^{m}r(j)^{-1}\right) + \frac{1}{m^2}\sum_{j=1}^{m}D_{z(j)}^2 r(j)^{-1}$$

P is the probability of obtaining a unit with full response, accepting that $E\left(r(j)^{-k}\right) \cong [E(r(j))]^{-k}$ we obtain

$$E\left(V\left(\bar{z}'_{(rss)}\right)\right) \cong \frac{\sigma_z^2}{nP} - \frac{1}{nmP}\sum_{j=1}^{m}D_{z(j)}^2, n = mr$$

Then $E(k^{-1}) \cong [E(k)]^{-1} = nP$ and the expected gain in accuracy due to the use of RSS is

$$E(G(\bar{y}_k, \bar{y}'_{(rss)})) \cong \frac{1}{nmP}\sum_{j=1}^{m}D_{z(j)}^2$$

Samawi and Muttlak (1996) developed estimation of a ratio. The RSS counterpart estimator of the population ratio is $r_{(rss)} = \frac{\bar{y}_{(rss)}}{\bar{x}_{(rss)}}$ and the ratio of the estimator of the mean is $\bar{y}_{r(rss)} = r_{(rss)}\mu_X$. Take the Taylor approximation

$$\bar{y}_{r(rss)} \cong \bar{y}_{(rss)} - Q_1\left(\bar{x}_{(rss)} - \mu_X\right) + Q_2\left(\bar{x}_{(rss)} - \mu_X\right)^2 - Q_3\left(\bar{x}_{(rss)} - \mu_X\right)\left(\bar{y}_{(rss)} - \mu_Y\right)$$

where $Q_1 = \frac{\mu_Y}{\mu_X}$, $Q_2 = \frac{\mu_Y}{\mu_X^2}$ and $Q_3 = \frac{1}{\mu_X}$. Using the first order approximation

$$E\left(\bar{y}_{r(rss)}\right) \cong E\left(\bar{y}_{(rss)}\right) - Q_1 E\left(\bar{x}_{r(rss)} - \mu_X\right) = \mu_Y$$

The MSE is approximated considering the Taylor Series with terms $O(n^{-1})$ by

$$MSE\left(\bar{y}_{(rss)}\right) \cong Var\left(\bar{y}_{(rss)}\right) + Q_2^2 Var\left(\bar{x}_{(rss)}\right) - 2Q_1 Cov\left(\bar{x}_{(rss)}, \bar{y}_{(rss)}\right),$$

where $Cov\left(\bar{x}_{(rss)}, \bar{y}_{(rss)}\right) = E\left(\bar{x}_{(rss)} - \bar{X}\right)\left(\bar{y}_{(rss)} - \bar{Y}\right)$.

Bouza and Al-Omari (2011b, c) assumed that the ranking is performed on a known variable A which allows to rank X and Y. Using RSS and the structure of the estimators of the classes we have the RSS-classes characterized by

$$\bar{y}_{KC1(rss)} = \frac{\bar{y}'_{(rss)} + b(\mu_X - \bar{x}'_{(rss)})}{\bar{x}_{(rss)}}\mu_X$$

$$\bar{y}_{KC2(rss)} = \frac{\bar{y}'_{(rss)} + b(\mu_X - \bar{x}'_{(rss)})}{\bar{x}'_{(rss)}}\mu_X$$

$$\bar{y}_{KC3(rss)} = \frac{\bar{y}'_{(rss)} + b(\bar{x}_{(rss)} - \bar{x}'_{(rss)})}{\bar{x}'_{(rss)}}\bar{x}_{(rss)}$$

Proposition 4.1 The results of the RSS versions of Kadilar and Cingi (2008) estimators are

1. $\bar{y}_{KC1(rss)}$ has the Expected Mean Squared Error (EMSC)

$$
\begin{aligned}
E\left(\text{MSE}\left(\bar{y}_{KC1(rss)}\right)\right) &= M\left(\bar{y}_{KC1(rss)}\right) \\
&\cong \frac{\sigma_Y^2}{nP} + \frac{(R^2 - B^2)\sigma_X^2}{n} \\
&\quad - \frac{1}{n^2}\left(\frac{1}{P}\sum_{j=1}^{m} D_{Y(j)}^2 + (R^2 - B^2)\sum_{j=1}^{m} D_{X(j)}^2\right)
\end{aligned}
$$

and its expected bias is $\text{EB}\left(\bar{y}_{KC1(rss)}\right) \cong \frac{\mu_Y}{nP\,\mu_X^2}\left(\sigma_X^2 - \frac{\sum_{j=1}^{m} D_{X(j)}^2}{m}\right)$.

2. $\bar{y}_{KC2(rss)}$ has the EMSE

$$
\begin{aligned}
M\left(\bar{y}_{KC2(rss)}\right) &\cong \frac{\sigma_Y^2}{nP} + \frac{R^2\sigma_x^2 - B^2\sigma_{xy}}{nP} \\
&\quad - \frac{1}{nmP}\left(\sum_{j=1}^{m} D_{Y(j)}^2 + R^2\sum_{j=1}^{m} D_{X(j)}^2 - \sum_{j=1}^{m} D_{X(j)Y(j)}\right)
\end{aligned}
$$

where $D_{X(j)Y(j)} = \left(\mu_{X_{(j)}} - \mu_X\right)\left(\mu_{Y_{(j)}} - \mu_Y\right)$. The expected bias is

$$
\text{EB}\left(\bar{y}_{KC2(rss)}\right) = \frac{\mu_Y}{nP\,\mu_X^2}\left(\sigma_X^2 - \frac{\sum_{j=1}^{m} D_{X(j)}^2}{m}\right).
$$

3. $\bar{y}_{KC3(rss)}$ has the EMSE

$$
M\left(\bar{y}_{KC3(rss)}\right) \cong \frac{\sigma_Y^2}{nP} + \frac{(R+B)^2\sigma_x^2 - 2(R+b)\sigma_{xy}}{nP} - \varpi
$$

$$
\varpi = \frac{1}{nmP}\left((R+B)^2\sum_{j=1}^{m} D_{X(j)}^2 - 2(R+B)\sum_{j=1}^{m} D_{X(j)}^2 - \sum_{j=1}^{m} D_{X(j)Y(j)}\right)
$$

The expected bias is

$$
\text{EB}\left(\bar{y}_{KC3(rss)}\right) = \frac{\mu_Y}{nP\,\mu_X}\left(\sigma_{xy} - \frac{-\sum_{j=1}^{m} D_{X(j)Y(j)}}{m}\right)
$$

Proof From the results derived for $\bar{y}_{KC1}$ using the properties of RSS estimators we have that

$$M\left(\bar{y}_{KC1(rss)}\right) \cong \frac{\sigma_Y^2}{nP} + \frac{(R^2 - B^2)\sigma_X^2}{n} - \frac{1}{n^2}\left(\frac{1}{P}\sum_{j=1}^{m} D_{Y(j)}^2 + (R^2 - B^2)\sum_{j=1}^{m} D_{X(j)}^2\right)$$

As $E(C_{x(rss)}^2) \cong \frac{1}{nP\,\mu_X^2}\left(\sigma_X^2 - \frac{\sum_{j=1}^{m} D_{X(j)}^2}{m}\right)$ substituting

$$EB\left(\bar{y}_{KC1(rss)}\right) \cong \frac{\mu_Y}{nP\,\mu_X^2}\left(\sigma_X^2 - \frac{\sum_{j=1}^{m} D_{X(j)}^2}{m}\right)$$

Similarly we obtain the results stated for $\bar{y}_{KC2(rss)}$ $\square$
and $\bar{y}_{KC3(rss)}$.

From these results are derived that, $\bar{y}_{KC1(rss)}$ is more accurate $\bar{y}_{KC1}$ if $R^2 < B^2$. For $\bar{y}_{KC2(rss)}$ we have that it is more accurate whenever

$$\sum_{j=1}^{m} D_{Y(j)}^2 + R^2 \sum_{j=1}^{m} D_{X(j)}^2 > \sum_{j=1}^{m} D_{X(j)}D_{Y(j)}$$

This relationship is valid generally. In the particular case in which the linear model $Y = BX + e$ holds it is reduced to

$$R^2 \sum_{j=1}^{m} D_{X(j)}^2 > \sum_{j=1}^{m} D_{X(j)}D_{Y(j)} \cong B \sum_{j=1}^{m} D_{X(j)}^2.$$

$\bar{y}_{KC3(rss)}$ is more accurate than its srs counterpart when $\varpi > 0$. If Y can be expressed by $Y = BX + e$ this condition holds when $R(B - 2) + B(B^2 + 2RB - 3) > 0$.

The corresponding RSS version of Singh and Horn (2000) estimator is

$$\bar{y}_{SH(rss)} = \alpha\bar{y}'_{(rss)} + \frac{(1 - \alpha)\bar{y}'_{(rss)}}{\bar{x}'_{(rss)}}\bar{x}_{(rss)}$$

Its behavior is characterized in the following proposition.

Proposition 4.2 The expected bias of $\bar{y}_{SH(rss)}$ is approximated by

$$EB(\bar{y}_{SH(rss)}) \cong \frac{(1 - \alpha_0)\mu_Y}{nP}\left(\frac{\sigma_X^2}{\mu_X^2} - \rho\frac{\sigma_X\sigma_Y}{\mu_X\mu_Y} - \left(\frac{\sum_{j=1}^{m} D_{X(j)}^2}{m\mu_X^2} + \frac{\sum_{j=1}^{m} D_{Y(j)}^2}{m\mu_Y^2} - 2\frac{\sum_{j=1}^{m} D_{X(j)Y(j)}}{m\mu_X\mu_Y}\right)\right),$$

$$\alpha_0 = 1 - \rho\frac{C_Y}{C_X}, C_Z = \frac{\sigma_Z}{\mu_Z}, Z = X, Y$$

Its EMSE is $M(\bar{y}_{SH(rss)}) \cong M(\bar{y}_k) - (\varpi_1 + \varpi_2)$

where

$$\varpi_1 = \frac{R^2}{nmP} \left(\frac{\sum_{j=1}^{m} D_{X(j)}^2}{m\mu_X^2} + \frac{\sum_{j=1}^{m} D_{Y(j)}^2}{m\mu_Y^2} - 2\frac{\sum_{j=1}^{m} D_{X(j)Y(j)}}{m\mu_X\mu_Y} \right)$$

$$\varpi_2 = \frac{R^2}{nP} \left(1 - \frac{\rho}{R} \left(\sqrt{\frac{\sigma_Y^2 - \sum_{j=1}^{m} \frac{D_{X(j)}^2}{m}}{\sigma_X^2 - \sum_{j=1}^{m} \frac{D_{Y(j)}^2}{m}}} \right) \right) \left(\sigma_X^2 - \frac{\sum_{j=1}^{m} D_{X(j)}^2}{m} \right)$$

Proof It follows using the same procedure as in the previous proposition: setting the results of the SRSWR case and using the properties of the RSS estimators.□

Note that the first term at the right-hand side of $M(\bar{y}_{SH(rss)})$ is the error of the srswr ratio estimator. Under the linear regression model $Y = BX + e$ we have that $\varpi_1 = \frac{B^2}{nmP} \left((B-1) \frac{\sum_{j=1}^{m} D_{X(j)}^2}{m\mu_X^2} \right)$, which is positive if $B > 1$. On the other hand $\varpi_2 = \frac{B^2}{nP} (1 - \rho B) \left(\sigma_X^2 - \frac{\sum_{j=1}^{m} D_{X(j)}^2}{m} \right)$. As $\rho B > 0$ the first within brackets term cannot be negative, hence the RSS estimator is always more accurate than its srswr version.

The RSS counterpart of $\bar{y}_{SD(rss)}$ is

$$\bar{y}_{SD(rss)} = \bar{y}'_{(rss)} \left(\frac{\bar{x}}{\bar{x}_{(rss)}} \right)^{\gamma_0}$$

Proposition 4.3 The expected bias of $\bar{y}_{SD(rss)}$ is

$$EB(\bar{y}_{SD(rss)}) \cong \frac{\mu_Y \left(\alpha(\alpha-1)C_X^2 - \alpha C_X C_Y \right)}{nP}$$
$$- \frac{1}{nP} \left(\frac{\alpha(\alpha-1)\sum_{j=1}^{m} D_{X(j)}^2}{2\mu_X^2} - \frac{\sum_{j=1}^{m} D_{X(j)Y(j)}}{\mu_X \mu_Y} \right)$$

The approximated expected MSE is given by

$$M(\bar{y}_{SD(rss)}) \cong M(\bar{y}_k) - \left(\frac{\sigma_X^2(B-R)^2 - R^2 G(KC1, RSS)}{nP} \right)$$
$$- \frac{1}{nP} \left(\frac{(B-R)^2 \sum_{j=1}^{m} D_{X(j)}^2}{m} \right)$$

Proof We omit it for same reasons used in the previous propositions.   □

Remark 4.4 Note that again the gain in accuracy may be negative but if $Y = BX + e$ the proposed estimator is more accurate than $\bar{y}_{SD}$.

4.4 Imputation in Median RSS

4.4.1 Some Quotations

We will consider the behavior of the RSS median estimator, see Chap. 2. The srswr model was first proposed by Muttlak (1997). Some other contribution in median estimstion are Jemain and Al-Omari (2006). For an economy in the notations we will drop be subindex Y in the notation of the mean and variance when there is no possible confusion.

The use of subsampling for obtaining information from the non-respondents was presented in Chap. 3. We will consider the use of imputation procedures.

4.4.2 Mean Imputation

Let us consider that there are non-responses. First, we will study the effect of imputation of the missing observations.

The first imputation method to be analyzed is the mean substitution. Take n odd

$$Y^*_{(i:\text{med})\text{mI}(1)} = \begin{cases} Y_{(i:\text{med})m} & \text{if a response is obtained} \\ \frac{1}{n(1)} \sum Y_{(i:\text{med})m} \; w(i:m) & \text{otherwiseas} \end{cases}$$

where $w(i{:}m)$ is a Bernoulli random variable with parameter $Q = 1-P$, P is the probability of response. Hence if the number of responses is $n(1)$

$$\sum_{i=1}^{n} w(i:m) = n(2).$$

Proposition 4.5 Taking $n(2) = n-n(1)$, the imputation estimator and $E(a/b) \cong E(a)/E(b)$

$$\mu_{\{\text{rss}\}\text{medI}(1)} = \mu_{I(1o)}$$
$$= \frac{\sum_{i=1}^{n(1)} \sum_{m=1}^{r} Y_{(i:\text{med})m} + \sum_{i=1}^{n} \frac{w(i:m)}{n(1)} \sum_{m=1}^{r} \left(\sum_{j=1}^{n(1)} Y*_{(j:\text{med})m} \right)_i}{nr}$$

If n is odd:

$$E\left(\mu_{I(1o)}\right) = \mu_{\left(\frac{n+1}{2}\right)}, \text{ and } E\left(V\left(\mu_{I(1o)}\right)\right) \frac{\left(nP + \frac{Q}{P}\right)\sigma^2_{\left(\frac{n+1}{2}\right)}}{n^2 r}$$

If n is even

$$\mu_{I(1e)} = \frac{\sum_{i=1}^{n(1)} \sum_{m=1}^{r} Y_{(i:\text{med})m} + \sum_{i=1}^{n} \frac{w(((1)i:m)}{n(11)} \sum_{m=1}^{r} \left(\sum_{j=1}^{n(11)} Y*_{(j:\text{med})m}\right)_i}{2nr}$$

$$+ \frac{\sum_{i=1}^{n} \frac{w(((2)i:m)}{n(11)} \sum_{m=1}^{r} \left(\sum_{j=1}^{n(11)} Y*_{(j:\text{med})m}\right)_i}{2nr}$$

with expectation $E\left(\mu_{I(1e)}\right) = \frac{\mu_{\left(\frac{n}{2}\right)} + \mu_{\left(\frac{n}{2}+1\right)}}{2}$ and expected variance

$$EV(\mu_{I(1e)}) \cong \frac{1}{4n^2 r}\left(\left(nP(1) + \frac{Q(1)}{P(1)}\right)\sigma^2_{\left(\frac{n}{2}\right)} + \left(nP(2) + \frac{Q(2)}{P(2)}\right)\sigma^2_{\left(\frac{n}{2}+1\right)}\right)$$

Accepting that $w((h)i:m)$, $h = 1, 2$, is a Bernoulli random variable with parameter $Q(h) = 1 - P(h)$, $P(h)$ is the probability of response in the h-th set of samples.

Proof Consider n odd

$$E\left(\mu_{I(1o)}\right) = \frac{\sum_{i=1}^{n(1)} \sum_{m=1}^{r} \mu_{\left(\frac{n+1}{2}\right)} + \sum_{i=1}^{n(2)} \sum_{m=1}^{r} \mu_{\left(\frac{n+1}{2}\right)}}{nr} = \mu_{\left(\frac{n+1}{2}\right)}$$

The conditional variance is

$$V\left(\mu_{I(1o)}\right) = \frac{\sum_{i=1}^{n(1)} \sum_{m=1}^{r} V(Y_{(i:\text{med})m}) + \sum_{i=1}^{n} w(i:m)^2 \sum_{m=1}^{r} V\left(\sum_{j=1}^{n(1)} \frac{Y_{(j:\text{med})m}}{n(1)}\right)_i}{(nr)^2}$$

$$= \frac{rn(1)\sigma^2_{\left(\frac{n+1}{2}\right)} + \frac{rn(2)\sigma^2_{\left(\frac{n+1}{2}\right)}}{n(1)}}{(nr)^2} = \frac{\left(n(1) + \frac{n(2)}{n(1)}\right)\sigma^2_{\left(\frac{n+1}{2}\right)}}{n^2 r}$$

and, accepting the approximation $E(a/b) \cong E(a)/E(b)$ the expected variance is

$$A = E(V\left(\mu_{I(1o)}\right))\frac{\left(nP + \frac{Q}{P}\right)\sigma^2_{\left(\frac{n+1}{2}\right)}}{n^2 r}$$

As in this case, the conditional expectation is not random and the error of the mean imputation median variance is equal to A.

When n is even we have to consider the no responses obtained in the two sets of samples.

$$Y^*_{(i:\text{med})mI(1)} = \begin{cases} Y_{(i:\text{med})m} & \text{if a response is obtained} \\ \frac{1}{n(11)}\sum_{j=1}^{n} Y_{(j:\text{med})m}w((1)j:m) & i \text{ does not respond and } i \leq n/2 \\ \frac{1}{n(12)}\sum_{j=1}^{n} Y_{(j:\text{med})m}w((2)j:m) & i \text{ does not respond and } i > n/2 \end{cases}$$

Now $w((h)i{:}m)$, $h = 1,2$, is a Bernoulli random variable with parameter $Q(h) = 1-P(h)$, $P(h)$ is the probability of response in the h-th set of samples. Hence if the number of responses are $n(1\ h)$, $h = 1, 2$, $n(1) = n(11) + n(12)$, and

$$\sum_{i=1}^{n} w((h)i : m) = n - n((h)1) = n(h2).$$

The imputation estimator proposed in this case is:

$$\mu_{\{rss\}medI(1)} = \mu_{I(1e)} = \frac{\sum_{i=1}^{n(1)} \sum_{m=1}^{r} Y_{(i:med)m} + I(1) + I(2)}{2nr}$$

where

$$I(1) = \sum_{i=1}^{n} \frac{w(((1)i : m)}{n(11)} \sum_{m=1}^{r} \left(\sum_{j=1}^{n(11)} Y*_{(j:med)m} \right)_i$$

$$I(2) = \sum_{i=1}^{n} \frac{w(((2)i : m)}{n(11)} \sum_{m=1}^{r} \left(\sum_{j=1}^{n(11)} Y*_{(j:med)m} \right)_i$$

We can divide $\mu_{I(1e)}$ as

$$\mu_{I(11)} = \frac{\sum_{i=1}^{n(11)} \sum_{m=1}^{r} Y_{(i:med)m} + I(1)}{2nr}$$

$$\mu_{I(12)} = \frac{\sum_{i=1}^{n(12)} \sum_{m=1}^{r} Y_{(i:med)m} + I(2)}{2nr}$$

The expectations of these terms are

$$E\left(\frac{\sum_{i=1}^{n(11)} \sum_{m=1}^{r} Y_{(i:med)m} + I(1)}{nr} \right)^* = \frac{(n(11) + n(21))\mu_{(\frac{n}{2})}}{n} = \frac{1}{2}\mu_{(\frac{n}{2})}$$

$$E\left(\frac{\sum_{i=1}^{n(12)} \sum_{m=1}^{r} Y_{(i:med)m} + I(2)}{nr} \right)^* = \frac{(n(12) + n(22))\mu_{(\frac{n}{2}+1)}}{n} = \frac{1}{2}\mu_{(\frac{n}{2}+1)}$$

Hence

$$E\left(\mu_{I(1e)} \right) = \frac{\mu_{(\frac{n}{2})} + \mu_{(\frac{n}{2}+1)}}{2}$$

Consequently, the variance of the conditional expectation is zero. The conditional variances are

$$V(\mu_{I(11)}) = \frac{1}{n^2 r}\left(n(11) + \frac{n(21)}{n(11)}\right)\sigma^2_{\left(\frac{n}{2}\right)}$$

$$V(\mu_{I(12)}) = \frac{1}{n^2 r}\left(n(12) + \frac{n(22)}{n(12)}\right)\sigma^2_{\left(\frac{n}{2}+1\right)}$$

Let us define $P(t)$ as the probability of obtaining a response of the statistics of order $n/2$ if $t = 1$ and $P(2)$ when $t = 2$ and the order is $1 + n/2$. Then

$$EV(\mu_{I(1e)}) \cong \frac{1}{4n^2 r}\left(\left(nP(1) + \frac{Q(1)}{P(1)}\right)\sigma^2_{\left(\frac{n}{2}\right)} + \left(nP(2) + \frac{Q(2)}{P(2)}\right)\sigma^2_{\left(\frac{n+2}{2}\right)}\right) \qquad \square$$

4.4.3 Ratio Imputation

Muttlak (2003) considered the use of quartiles for improving the estimation of the mean based on median RSS. Bouza and Al-Omari (2013) developed imputation procedures for the median RSS considering ratio imputation methods. Let μ_X be the population mean of the auxiliary variable X, and σ^2_x its population variance. X is a known variable and $\bar{x}$ is the mean of it in the sample. Consider the estimator $\bar{y}_{r(rss)} = \frac{\bar{y}_{(rss)}}{\bar{x}_{(rss)}}\mu_X$. A Taylor approximation is

$$\bar{y}_{r(rss)} \cong \bar{y}_{(rss)} - Q_1\left(\bar{x}_{(rss)} - \mu_X\right) + Q_2\left(\bar{x}_{(rss)} - \mu_X\right)^2 - Q_3\left(\bar{x}_{(rss)} - \mu_X\right)\left(\bar{y}_{(rss)} - \mu_Y\right)$$

where

$$Q_1 = \frac{\mu_Y}{\mu_X + q_i}, \quad Q_2 = \frac{\mu_Y}{\mu_X + q_i}\frac{1}{\mu_X + q_i}, \quad Q_3 = \frac{1}{\mu_X + q_i}\left(\bar{x}_{(rss)} - \mu_X\right)\left(\bar{y}_{(rss)} - \mu_Y\right)$$

Using these formulae it is derived that
The MSE approximated, considering the Taylor Series with terms $O(n^{-2})$ as a good approximation is

$$MSE(\bar{y}_{(rss)}) \cong Var(\bar{y}_{(rss)}) + Q_2^2 Var(\bar{x}_{(rss)}) - 2Q_1 Cov(\bar{x}_{(rss)}, \bar{y}_{(rss)})$$

where

$$Cov(\bar{x}_{(rss)}, \bar{y}_{(rss)}) = E(\bar{x}_{(rss)} - \mu_X)(\bar{y}_{(rss)} - \mu_Y)$$

These results are stated as follow:

Theorem 4.6 Bouza and Al-Omari (2013). Take the ratio of the RSS means as $r_{(rss)} = \frac{\bar{y}_{(rss)}}{\bar{x}_{(rss)}}$ and $\bar{y}_{r(rss)} = r_{(rss)}\mu_X$ as the estimated mean. Let Q_1 and Q_3 denote the known first and third quartiles of the distribution of X, respectively then

$$E(\bar{y}_{r(rss)}) \cong \mu_Y + Q_2 V(\bar{x}_{(rss)}) - Q_3 \text{Cov}(\bar{x}_{(rss)}, \bar{y}_{(rss)})$$

and

$$\text{MSE}(\bar{y}_{(rss)}) \cong \text{Var}(\bar{y}_{(rss)}) + Q_2^2 \text{Var}(\bar{x}_{(rss)}) - 2Q_1 \text{Cov}(\bar{x}_{(rss)}, \bar{y}_{(rss)}). \square$$

We will consider the median RSS estimator when there are missing observations. Define the Bernoulli random variable $w*(i{:}m)$ with probability of success $P(1)$. If we obtain a response at the ith-sample in the cycle m then $w(i{:}m) = 1$. The number of responses is

$$n(1) = \sum_{i=1}^{n} \sum_{m=1}^{r} w(i : m) = \sum_{i=1}^{n} r(i)$$

In the case of full response $r(i) = r$ for any i and $n(1) = n$.

When non-responses are present we propose to use the ratio of mean of the responses to Y to the mean in the sample of the auxiliary variable X. $r^*_{(rss)} = \dfrac{\mu^*_{Y_{(rss)}}}{\mu^*_{X_{(rss)}}}$ and $\bar{y}_{(rss)med(R)} = r^*_{(rss)}\mu_X$ are the ratio imputation estimator of the mean.

Proposition 4.7 Take $r^*_{(rss)} = \dfrac{\mu^*_{Y_{(rss)}}}{\mu^*_{X_{(rss)}}}$ and $\bar{y}_{(rss)med(R)} = r^*_{(rss)}\mu_X$ its expected value is

$$E(\bar{y}_{(rss)med(R)}) \cong \begin{cases} \mu_{Y_{\left(\frac{n+1}{2}\right)}} - Q_1 E(A(1)) + Q_2 E(A(2)) - Q_3 E(A(3)) & \text{if } n \quad \text{odd} \\[2ex] \dfrac{\mu_{Y_{\left(\frac{n}{2}\right)}} + \mu_{Y_{\left(\frac{n}{2}+1\right)}}}{2} - Q_1 E(A(1)) + Q_2 E(A(2)) - Q_3 E(A(3) & \text{if } n \quad \text{even} \end{cases}$$

where

$$E(A(1)) = \Delta_{X\left(\frac{n+1}{2}\right)}, \ E(A(2)) = \frac{\sigma^2_{X\left(\frac{n+1}{2}\right)}}{n^2 r^2} = \frac{\sigma^2_X}{n\,r} - \frac{(nr-1)\Delta^2_{X\left(\frac{n+1}{2}\right)}}{n\,r},$$

$$E(A(3)) = \text{Cov}(\bar{x}_{(rss)}, \bar{y}_{(rss)}) - \left(\mu_Y \Delta_{X\left(\frac{n+1}{2}\right)} + \mu_X \Delta_{Y\left(\frac{n+1}{2}\right)}\right)$$

and

$$EV\left(\mu^*_{Y_{(rss)}}\right) \cong \begin{cases} \dfrac{\sigma^2_{Y\left(\frac{n+1}{2}\cdot\right)}}{nP_{(1)}} & \text{if } n \text{ is odd} \\[2ex] \dfrac{\sigma^2_{Y\left(\frac{n}{2}\right)} + \sigma^2_{Y\left(\frac{n+2}{2}\right)}}{2nP_{(1)}} & \text{if } n \text{ is even} \end{cases}$$

Proof The mean of the responses to Y is

$$\mu^*_{Y_{(\mathrm{rss})}} = \frac{\sum_{i=1}^n \sum_{m=1}^r Y_{(i:\mathrm{med})m} w(i:m)}{n(1)}$$

Its expectation is given, for n odd, by:

$$E(\mu^*_{Y_{(\mathrm{rss})}}|s) = \frac{\sum_{i=1}^n \sum_{m=1}^r \mu_{Y_{\left(\frac{n+1}{2}\right)}} w(i:m)}{n(1)} = \mu_{Y_{\left(\frac{n+1}{2}\right)}}$$

and   hence   it   is   derived   that $E(\bar{y}_{(\mathrm{rss})\mathrm{med}(R)}) \cong \mu_{Y_{\left(\frac{n+1}{2}\right)}} - Q_1 E(A(1)) +$
$Q_2 E(A(2)) - Q_3 E(A(3))$.

For n even $\mu^*_{Y_{\mathrm{rss}}} = \frac{1}{2}\left(\sum_{i=1}^{\frac{n}{2}} \frac{\sum_{m=1}^r Y_{\left(i:\frac{n}{2}\right)m} w(i:m)}{n(11)} + \sum_{i=\frac{n}{2}+1}^n \frac{\sum_{m=1}^r Y_{\left(i:\frac{n}{2}+1\right)m} w(i:m)}{n(12)}\right)$ and

$n(1) = \sum_{i=1}^{\frac{n}{2}} \sum_{m=1}^r w(i:m) + \sum_{i=\frac{n}{2}+1}^n \sum_{m=1}^r w(i:m) = n(11) + n(12)$. Calculat-

ing the expected value we have that $EE\left(\mu^*_{Y_{\mathrm{rss}}}|s\right) = \frac{\mu_{Y_{\left(\frac{n}{2}\right)}} + \mu_{Y_{\left(\frac{n}{2}+1\right)}}}{2}$ and we derive that

$$E(\bar{y}_{(\mathrm{rss})\mathrm{med}(R)}) \cong \frac{\mu_{Y_{\left(\frac{n}{2}\right)}} + \mu_{Y_{\left(\frac{n}{2}+1\right)}}}{2} - Q_1 E(A(1)) + Q_2 E(A(2)) - Q_3 E(A(3))$$

The conditional variances of the terms of $\mu^*_{Y(\mathrm{rss})}$ for n even are

$$V(\mu^*_{Y_{(\mathrm{rss})}}|s) = \frac{1}{2}\left(\sum_{i=1}^{\frac{n}{2}} \frac{\sum_{m=1}^r V(Y_{\left(i:\frac{n}{2}\right)m}) w^2(i:m)}{n^2(11)} + \sum_{i=\frac{n}{2}+1}^n \frac{\sum_{m=1}^r V(Y_{\left(i:\frac{n}{2}+1\right)m}) w^2(i:m)}{n^2(12)}\right)$$

$$= \frac{1}{2}\left(\sigma^2_{Y_{\left(\frac{n}{2}\right)}} \sum_{i=1}^{\frac{n}{2}} \frac{\sum_{m=1}^r w^2(i:m)}{n^2(11)} + \sigma^2_{Y_{\left(\frac{n}{2}+1\right)}} \sum_{i=\frac{n}{2}+1}^n \frac{\sum_{m=1}^r w^2(i:m)}{n^2(12)}\right)$$

Then

$$E(V(\mu^*_{Y_{(\mathrm{rss})}}|s)) = \frac{\sigma^2_{Y_{\left(\frac{n}{2}\right)}} + \sigma^2_{Y_{\left(\frac{n}{2}+1\right)}}}{2nP(1)}$$

On the other hand

$$V(E(\mu^*_{Y_{(\mathrm{rss})}}|s)) = \frac{1}{4}\left(\mu^2_{Y_{\left(\frac{n}{2}\right)}} V\left(\sum_{i=1}^{\frac{n}{2}} \frac{\sum_{m=1}^r w(i:m)}{n(11)}\right) + \mu^2_{Y_{\left(\frac{n}{2}+1\right)}} V\left(\sum_{i=\frac{n}{2}+1}^n \frac{\sum_{m=1}^r w(i:m)}{n(12)}\right)\right) = 0$$

Hence

$$\varepsilon\left(\mu^*_{Y_{(rss)}}\right) = EV\left(\mu^*_{Y_{(rss)}}\right) \cong \begin{cases} \dfrac{\sigma^2_{Y_{\left(\frac{n+1}{2}:t\right)}}}{n\overline{P}_{(1)}} & \text{if } n \text{ is odd} \\[2ex] \Box \\ \dfrac{\sigma^2_{Y_{\left(\frac{n}{2}\right)}} + \sigma^2_{Y_{\left(\frac{n+2}{2}\right)}}}{2n\overline{P}_{(1)}} & \text{if } n \text{ is even} \end{cases}$$

4.5 Imputation Using Product-Type Estimators

Bouza (2008a) proposed an imputation procedure based on a product-type predictor of the non-respondents. The prediction of the mean of the non-respondents is:

$$\bar{y}^*_{2p} = \frac{\sum\limits_{i=1}^{n_2} \frac{x_i}{\mu_X}\bar{y}_1}{n_2}$$

for computing the mean of the missing observations. Mimicking the estimator developed for subsampling the non-respondent strata we propose

$$\bar{y}_{IC} = \frac{n_1\bar{y}_1 + n_2\bar{y}^*_{2p}}{n}$$

Due to the conditional independence between the subsamples we have that

$$E(E(\bar{y}_{IC}|s)) = E\left(\frac{n_1\mu_1 + n_2\frac{\mu_{1Y}\mu_{2X}}{\mu_X}}{n}\right) = W_1\mu_1 + W_2\frac{\mu_{1Y}\mu_{2X}}{\mu_X}$$

Its bias is

$$B(\bar{y}_{IC}) = W_2\left(\frac{\mu_{2X}\mu_{1Y}}{\mu_X} - \mu_{2Y}\right)$$

Hence if the population is balanced in the sense $\mu_{2X} \cong \mu_X$. The bias of $\bar{y}^*_{2p}$ is equal to the bias obtained when a srswr is the sampling design and the information provided by s_1 is used. Expressing $\bar{y}_{IC}$ as

$$\bar{y}_{IC} = \bar{y} + \frac{n_2}{n}\left(\bar{y}_{2p} - \bar{y}_2\right)$$

is easily derived that

$$V(E(\bar{y}_{IC}(s))) = \left(\frac{\mu_{1Y}\mu_{2X}}{\mu_X} - \mu_{1Y}\right)^2\frac{W_1W_2}{n}$$

The conditional variance of the estimator is

$$V(\bar{y}_{IC}|s) = V(\bar{y}|s) + \left(\frac{n_2}{n}\right)^2 V\left(\bar{y}_{2p}^* - \bar{y}_2|s\right)$$

because the cross term is equal to zero. The expectation of the first term is

$$E(V(\bar{y}|s)) = V(IC-1) = E\left(\frac{w_1^2\sigma_{1Y}^2 + w_2^2\sigma_{2Y}^2}{n^2}\right)$$

$$= \frac{(nW_1^2 + W_1 W_2)\sigma_{1Y}^2 + (nW_2^2 + W_1 W_2)\sigma_{2Y}^2}{n}$$

The expectation of the second term is

$$V\left(\bar{y}_{2p}^* - \bar{y}_2\{s\}\right) = V(\bar{y}*_{2p}\{s\}) + V(\bar{y}_2\{s\}) - 2\mathrm{Cov}(\bar{y}*_{2p}, \bar{y}_2\{s\})$$

Note that

$$V\left(\bar{y}_{2p}^*|s\right) = \frac{\sum_{i-1}^{n_2} E(x_i\bar{y}_1)^2 - \mu_{1Y}\mu_{2X}\mu_{2Y}}{n_2^2\mu_X^2}$$

As the subsamples are independent the first term in the numerator is the product of the expectation and is equal to

$$\eta(1) = \frac{(\mu_{2X}^2 + \sigma_{2X}^2)\left(\mu_{1Y}^2 + \frac{\sigma_{1Y}^2}{n_1}\right)}{n_2\mu_X^2}$$

The expectation of the other terms sum $-\mu_{1Y}\mu_{2X}$. Then the second term of (4.4) is given by

$$\left(\frac{n_2^2}{n}\right)^2 V\left(\bar{y}_{2p}^*|s\right) = \left(\frac{n_2}{n^2\mu_X^2}\right)\left(\mu_{1Y}^2\sigma_{2X}^2 + \mu_{1Y}^2\mu_{2X}^2 + \frac{\mu_{2X}^2\sigma_{1Y}^2}{n_1} + \frac{\mu_{1Y}^2\sigma_{2X}^2}{n_1}\right)$$

Hence the expectation of the second term in the conditional variance $V(\bar{y}_{IC}|s)$ is

$$V(IC-2) = \left(\frac{W_2}{n\,\mu_X^2}\right)(\mu_{1Y}^2\sigma_{2X}^2 + \mu_{1Y}^2\mu_{2X}^2) + \frac{\mu_{2X}^2\sigma_{1Y}^2 + \mu_{1Y}^2\sigma_{2X}^2}{n^2\mu_X^2}E\left(\frac{n_2}{n_1}\right)$$

Doing some algebraic arrangements we have that its expected value is

$$V^* \cong \frac{(nW_1^2 + W_1 W_2)\sigma_{1Y}^2 + (nW_2^2 + W_1 W_2)\sigma_{2Y}^2}{n} + \frac{W_2(\mu_{1Y}^2\sigma_{2X}^2 + \mu_{1Y}^2\mu_{2X}^2)}{n\mu_X^2}$$

$$+ \frac{W_2(\mu_{1X}^2\sigma_{1Y}^2 + \mu_{1Y}\sigma_{2X}^2)}{n^2 W_1\mu_X^2}$$

The expected variance second term of the srswr mean of the non-respondent subsample is equal to $V^{**} = E(n_2 \sigma_2^2 / n^2) = W_2 \sigma_2^2 / n$.

The development of the covariance term leads to accept that it is equal to zero. Then we can state now the following Lemma.

Proposition 4.8 The estimator $\bar{y}_{IC}$ is equivalent to $\bar{y}_1$ if the first order population balancedness $\mu_{2X} \cong \mu_X$. holds and its variance is approximately equal to

$$V_{IC} = \left(\frac{\mu_{2X}^2 \mu_{1Y}^2}{\mu_X} - \mu_{1Y} \right) \left(\frac{W_1 W_2}{n} \right)$$
$$+ \frac{(nW_1^2 + W_1 W_2)\sigma_{1Y}^2 + (nW_2^2 + (W_1 + 1)W)\sigma_{2Y}^2}{n} + \frac{W_2(\mu_{1Y}^2 \sigma_{2X}^2 + \mu_{1Y}^2 \mu_{2X}^2)}{n\mu_X^2}$$

when $n \to \infty$ and the second order regularity condition $E\left(n_2^t / n_1^q\right) \cong E(n_2^t / E(/n_1^q)), t = 1, \ldots 4, h = 1, \ldots, 4$ is satisfied.

Proof The first result is obtained by using the balance condition posed and simplifying the derived bias.

Take

$$V(E(\bar{y}_{IC}|s)) + V^*$$

Assuming that $E\left(n_2^t / n_1^q\right) \cong E(n_2^t / E(/n_1^q)), t = 1, \ldots 4, h = 1, \ldots, 4$ holds that we have for n sufficiently large for accepting the terms of order $O(n^{-2})$ in the variance are negligible and we have the stated result. □

In many occasions the interest of the results is not only to estimate the mean but to predict the response of the individual non-responses. The estimator proposed is not longer a solution. Proposed the use of a ratio imputation method for the missing values of the variable Y in the non-response item 'i':

$$y_{il} = \left(\frac{\bar{y}_1}{\bar{x}_1} \right) x_i$$

Liu et al. (2006) proposed using

$$y_{ill} = \left(\frac{1}{n_1} \sum_{j=1}^{n_1} \frac{y_j}{x_j} \right) x_i$$

We will use the auxiliary information provided by X using the product estimation principle. The result is the imputed value

$$y_i^{**} = \frac{\bar{y}_1 \bar{x}_1}{\mu_X} x_i$$

for the missing observation i. Its expectation is $E\left(y_i^{**}|s\right) = \left(\frac{\sigma_{1XY} \bar{x}_1}{n_1} + \mu_{1X} \mu_{1Y} \right) \frac{\mu_{2X}}{\mu_X}$.

Hence if the condition $C(n) : E(n_2^t/n_1^q) \cong E(n_2^t / E(/n_1^q)$, $t = 1, \ldots 4$, $h = 1, \ldots, 4$ is accepted the mean of the imputed values has as an approximated expected value

$$\mathrm{EE}\left(\frac{\sum_{i=1}^{n_2} y_i^{**}}{n_2} \,\middle|\, s\right) \equiv \left(\frac{\sigma_{1XY}\bar{x}_1}{nW_1} + \mu_{1X}\mu_{1Y}\right)\frac{\mu_{2X}}{\mu_X}$$

For improving the simplicity in the reasoning let us consider the estimator of μ_Y

$$\bar{y}_{IS} = \frac{n_1\bar{y}_1 + n_2\bar{y}_{2p}^{**}}{n}$$

using the expression

$$\bar{y}_{IS} = \bar{y} + \frac{n_2(\bar{y}_{2p}^{**} - \bar{y}_2)}{n}$$

Its conditional mean is given by

$$E(\bar{y}_{IS}|s) = \frac{w_1\mu_{1Y} + w_2\mu_{2Y}}{n} + \frac{n_2\left(\frac{\mu_{2X}\sigma_{1XY}}{n_1\mu_X} + \frac{\mu_{1X}\mu_{1Y}\mu_{2X}}{\mu_X} - \mu_{2X}\right)}{n}$$

Calculating the expected value of this last expression we have that

$$E(E(\bar{y}_{IS}|s)) = \mu_Y + W_2\left(\frac{\mu_{1X}\mu_{1Y}\mu_{2X}}{\mu_X} - \mu_{2X}\right) + \frac{\mu_{2X}\sigma_{1XY}}{n\mu_X}E\left(\frac{n_2}{n_1}\right)$$

The two last terms are equal to the bias of $\bar{y}_{IS}$. Note that that it is considerably larger than the bias of the combined product estimator. If $C(n)$ is accepted we have an approximation to the expectation of $\bar{y}_{IS}$ given by

$$E(E(\bar{y}_{IS}|s)) \equiv \mu_Y + W_2\left(\frac{\mu_{1X}\mu_{1Y}\mu_{2X}}{\mu_X} - \mu_{2X}\right) + \frac{W_2\mu_{2X}\sigma_{1XY}}{nW_1\mu_X}$$

It is also larger than the bias of $\bar{y}_{IC}$.

The calculation of error of the imputed mean using the separated principle is very cumbersome. We will give the main results in the sequel.

Accepting that $C(n)$ is valid

$$V(E(\bar{y}_{IS}|s)) \cong \frac{W_1W_2\left(\mu_{1Y}^2 + \mu_{2Y}^2\right)}{n} + \left(\frac{\mu_{2X}\sigma_{1XY}}{n\mu_X}\right)^2 = V(1IPS)$$

Take

$$V(\bar{y}_{IS}|s) = V(\bar{y}|s) + \left(\frac{n_2}{n}\right)^2 V(\bar{y}_{2P}^{**} - \bar{y}_2|s) + 2\left(\frac{n_2}{n}\right)\mathrm{Cov}\left(\bar{y}, (\bar{y}_{2P}^{**} - \bar{y}_2|s)\right)$$

The first term is equal to zero and

$$V_{2P|s} = V\big((\bar{y}_{2P}^{**} - \bar{y}_2|s)\big) = E(\bar{y}_{2P}^{**}|s)^2 E(\bar{y}_2|s)^2 - 2E(\bar{y}_{2P}^{**}\bar{y}_2|s) - \big(E(\bar{y}_{2P}^{**} - \bar{y}_2|s)\big)^2$$

We computed the terns and arranged the similar terms. Afterwards the unconditional expectation was calculated. Assuming that the regularity conditions $C(n)$ and $C(W) : W_2^t \cong 0$, for $t \geq 3$ hold we have that

$$EV_{2P|s} \cong V(1ps) + V(2ps) + V(3ps) + V(4ps) = V(2IPS)$$

where

$$V(1ps) \cong W_2\left(2\mu_{1X}\mu_{1Y}\mu_{2X}\mu_{2Y} + \mu_{1X}\mu_{1Y}\mu_{2X}\mu_Y + \frac{\sigma_{2X}^2}{n} + \frac{\mu_{1X}\mu_{1Y}\sigma_{2XY}}{n\mu_X}\right)$$

$$V(2ps) \cong W_2^2\left(\left(\frac{\mu_{1X}\mu_{1Y}\mu_{2X}}{\mu_X}\right)^2 + W_1\mu_{2Y}^2 - \frac{2(\mu_{1X}\mu_{1Y} + \mu_{1X}\mu_{1Y}\mu_{2X}\mu_Y)}{nW_1\mu_X}\right)$$

$$V(3ps) \cong \left(\frac{\sigma_{1XY}\mu_{21Y}}{\mu_X}\right)^2 + \frac{2W_2\sigma_{1XY}\mu_{1X}\mu_{1Y}\mu_{2X}^2}{nw_1\mu_X^2}$$

$$V(4ps) \cong \frac{W_1(\sigma_{1XY} + \mu_{1X}\mu_{1Y}\mu_{2X})}{n\mu_X} + \left(\frac{\mu_{1X}\mu_{1Y}\mu_{2X}\mu_{2Y}}{n\mu_X}\right)$$

Let us fixe the behavior of the separate imputation product estimator.

Proposition 4.9 The estimator $\bar{y}_{IS}$ is biased and $\bar{y}_1$ is preferred in terms of the bias and variance.

Proof Comparing the biases the first affirmation is evident. On the other hand, as the approximate variance of $\bar{y}_{IS}$ is $V(ISP) = V(1IPS) + V(2IPS)$, the second result is obtained because it is larger than the variance of $\bar{y}_1$. □

4.6 Imputation in LRSS

4.6.1 Modeling the Non-responses

Al-Nasser (2007) considered that in common practice, some of the units cannot be measured. Assume that the non responses are generated at random (MAR mechanism). For $1 \leq i \leq k$ our information allows to compute

$$T_{(k+1)} = \sum_{i=1}^{k}\sum_{j=1}^{r} Y_{i(k+1)j}\alpha(i,j)$$

where

$$\alpha(i,j) = \begin{cases} 1 \text{ if a response is obtained for the unit } i \text{ at the cycle } j \\ 0 \text{ if not} \end{cases}$$

is a Bernoulli random variable with parameter W.

The number of responses of the corresponding units is $r(1|k) = \sum_{i=1}^{k} \sum_{j=1}^{r} \alpha(i,j)$ and $r^*(1|k) = r - r(1|k)$ is the number of missing responses.

4.6.2 The Mean Substitution

Under this model and the use of the imputations by the mean substitution method, we redefine the measurements for $1 \leq i \leq k$ as

$$Y^*_{i(k+1)j} = \begin{cases} Y_{i(k+1)j} & \text{if a response is obtained for } i-\text{th ordered unit at cycle } j \\ \frac{T_{(k+1)}}{r(i|k)} & \text{if non response is obtained for the } i-\text{th ordered unit at cycle } j \end{cases}$$

and $r(i|k)$ as the number of responding units associated to the i-th os.
    For $k+1 \leq m - k - 1$

$$Y^*_{i(i)j} = \begin{cases} Y_{i(i)j} & \text{if a response is obtained for } i\text{-th ordered unit at cycle } j \\ \frac{T_{(i)}}{r(2|k)} & \text{if non response is obtained for the } i\text{-th ordered unit at cycle } j \end{cases}$$

$$T_{(i)} = \sum_{j=1}^{r} Y_{i(i)j} \alpha(i,j)$$

In this case $r(2|k) = \sum_{i=k+1}^{m-k-1} \sum_{j=1}^{r} \alpha(i,j)$ and we have $r^*(2|k) = r - r(1|k)$ non responses.
    In the third set of units we define

$$Y^*_{i(m-k)j} = \begin{cases} Y_{i(m-k)j} & \text{if a response is obtained for } i-\text{th ordered unit at cycle } j \\ \frac{T_{(m-k)}}{r(3|k)} & \text{if non response is obtained for the } i-\text{th ordered unit at cycle } j \end{cases}$$

where $r(3|k)$ is the number of responses and $r^*(3|k) = r - r(3|k)$ of non responses and

$$T_{(m-k)} = \sum_{i=1}^{k} \sum_{j=1}^{r} Y_{i(m-k)j} \alpha(i,j)$$

Proposition 4.11 Bouza (2012): Take

$$\bar{y}_{\text{LRSS}(M)} = \frac{\sum_{j=1}^{r}\left(\sum_{i=1}^{k} Y_{*i(k+1)j} + \sum_{i=k+1}^{m-k} Y_{*i(i)j} + \sum_{i=m-k+1}^{m} Y_{*i(m-k)j}\right)}{mr} = \frac{T(1)+T(2)*T(3)}{mr}$$ its

expectation is

$$E(\bar{y}_{\text{LRSS}(M)}) = \frac{k\left[\mu_{(k+1)} + \mu_{(m-k)}\right] + \sum_{i=k+1}^{m-k} \mu_{(i)}}{m}$$

Its variance is given by

$$V(\bar{y}_{\text{LRSS}(M)})$$
$$= \frac{\sum_{i=1}^{k} \sigma_{(k+1)}^2\left(r(1|k) + \frac{r^*(1|k)}{r(1|k)}\right) + \sum_{i=k+1}^{m-k} \sigma_{(i)}^2\left(r(2|k) + \frac{1}{r^*(2|k)}\right) + \sum_{i=1}^{k} \sigma_{(m-k)}^2\left(r(3|k) + \frac{r^*(3|k)}{r(3|k)}\right)}{(mr)^2}$$

Proof The expectations with respect to RSS procedure are

$$E(T(1)) = \sum_{i=1}^{k}\left(\sum_{j\in s(1,R)} \mu_{(k+1)} + \sum_{j\in s(2,NR)} \mu_{(k+1)}\right) = kr\mu_{(k+1)}$$

$$E(T(2)) = \sum_{i=k+1}^{m-k}\left(\sum_{j\in s(2,R)} \mu_{(i)} + \sum_{j\in s(2,NR)} \mu_{(i)}\right) = \sum_{i=k+1}^{m-k} r\mu_{(i)}$$

$$E(T(3)) = \sum_{i=m-k-1}^{m}\left(\sum_{j\in s(3,R)} \mu_{(m-k)} + \sum_{j\in s(3,NR)} \mu_{(m-k)}\right) = kr\mu_{(m-k)}$$

Then we have that $E(\bar{y}_{\text{LRSS}(M)}) = \frac{k\left[\mu_{(k+1)}+\mu_{(m-k)}\right]+\sum_{i=k+1}^{m-k} \mu_{(i)}}{m}$.

Let us consider the conditional variance of this estimator. Due to the independence

$$V(T(1)) = \sum_{i=1}^{k}\left(\sum_{j\in s(1,R)} \sigma_{(k+1)}^2 + \sum_{j\in s(2,NR)} \frac{\sigma_{(k+1)}^2}{r(1|k)}\right) = \sum_{i=1}^{k} \sigma_{(k+1)}^2\left(r(1|k) + \frac{r^*(1|k)}{r(1|k)}\right)$$

$$V(T(2)) = \sum_{i=k+1}^{m-k}\left(\sum_{j\in s(2,R)} \sigma_{(i)}^2 + \sum_{j\in s(2,NR)} \frac{r(i)\sigma_{(i)}^2}{(r^*(2|k))^2}\right) = \sum_{i=k+1}^{m-k} \sigma_{(i)}^2\left(r(2|k) + \frac{1}{r^*(2|k)}\right)$$

$$V(T(3)) = \sum_{i=m-k-1}^{m}\left(\sum_{j\in s(3,R)} \sigma_{(m-k)}^2 + \sum_{j\in s(3,NR)} \frac{\sigma_{(m-k)}^2}{r(3|k)}\right) = \sum_{i=1}^{k} \sigma_{(m-k)}^2\left(r(3|k) + \frac{r^*(3|k)}{r(3|k)}\right)$$

Hence

$$V(\bar{y}_{\text{LRSS}(M)})$$
$$= \frac{\sum_{i=1}^{k} \sigma_{(k+1)}^2\left(r(1|k) + \frac{r^*(1|k)}{r(1|k)}\right) + \sum_{i=k+1}^{m-k} \sigma_{(i)}^2\left(r(2|k) + \frac{1}{r^*(2|k)}\right) + \sum_{i=1}^{k} \sigma_{(m-k)}^2\left(r(3|k) + \frac{r^*(3|k)}{r(3|k)}\right)}{(mr)^2}$$

Remark 4.12 Our proposal leads to an estimator which is unbiased if the distribution is symmetric.

This result fixes that $V(E(\bar{y}_{\text{LRSS}(M)})) = 0$.

Substituting the $os's$ variances in this expression the unconditional variance can be written as

$$V\left(\bar{y}_{\mathrm{LRSS}(M)}\right) = \frac{\sigma^2}{mr} - \beta$$

taking $\beta = B(1) + B(2) + B(3)$ where $B(1) = \dfrac{k\Delta^2_{(k+1)}\left(r(1|k)+\frac{r^*(1|k)}{r(1|k)}\right)}{(mr)^2}$, $B(2) =$

$\dfrac{\sum_{i=1}^{k} + \sum_{i=k+1}^{m-k} \Delta^2_{(i)}\left(r(2|k)+\frac{1}{r^*(2|k)}\right)}{(mr)^2}$ and $B(3) = \dfrac{\Delta^2_{(m-k)}\left(r(3|k)+\frac{r^*(3|k)}{r(3|k)}\right)}{(mr)^2}$..

Remark 4.13 Note that if for $t = 1,\ 2,\ 3$ we have $\left(r(t|k) + \frac{r^*(t|k)}{r(t|k)}\right) = r$ then $V\left(\bar{y}_{\mathrm{LRSS}(M)}\right) = V(\bar{y}_{\mathrm{LRSS}})$ which holds when there are not NR.

4.6.3 Ratio Imputation

Let us consider the ratio imputation method. Take X as the auxiliary variable used for ranking Y and $\overline{X}$ as its population mean. The proposed L-RSS ratio is

$$R(\mathrm{LRSS}) = \frac{\sum_{j=1}^{r}\left(\sum_{i=1}^{k} Y_{i(k+1)j} + \sum_{i=k+1}^{m-k} Y_{i(i)j} + \sum_{i=m-k+1}^{m} Y_{i(m-k)j}\right)}{\sum_{j=1}^{r}\left(\sum_{i=1}^{k} X_{i(k+1)j} + \sum_{i=k+1}^{m-k} X_{i(i)j} + \sum_{i=m-k+1}^{m} X_{i(m-k)j}\right)} = \frac{t(Y)}{t(X)}$$

The estimation of the mean of Y based on this ratio is given by

$$\bar{y}_{R(\mathrm{LRSS})} = \overline{X} R(\mathrm{LRSS})$$

Following the usual approach used to analyze the ratio estimation defining $\frac{t(Z)}{mr} = z(\mathrm{LRSS})$ and $R = \mu/\overline{X}$

$$R(\mathrm{LRSS}) = R + \frac{\bar{y}(\mathrm{LRSS}) - R\bar{x}(\mathrm{LRSS})}{\overline{X}}\left(1 - \frac{\bar{x}(\mathrm{LRSS}) - \overline{X}}{\overline{X}}\right)$$

Taking $\Delta_{X(j)} = \overline{X}_{(j)} - \overline{X}$ we have that

$$A(\mathrm{LRSS}) = E(\bar{y}(\mathrm{LRSS}) - R\bar{x}(\mathrm{LRSS}))$$
$$= \frac{k\left[\left(\Delta_{(k+1)} - R\Delta_{X(k+1)}\right) + \left(\Delta_{(m-k)} - R\Delta_{X(m-k)}\right)\right] + \sum_{i=k+1}^{m-k}\left(\Delta_{(i)} - R - R\Delta_{X(i)}\right)}{mr}$$

Using the Taylor Series expansion the bias of this estimator is approximately

$$B(\bar{y}(\mathrm{LRSS})) \cong A(\mathrm{LRSS}) + B(\mathrm{LRSS}) + C(\mathrm{LRSS})$$

$$B(\mathrm{LRSS}) = \frac{R\left(\frac{\sigma^2_x}{mr}\right) + \frac{k}{m^2 r}[\Delta^2_{X(k+1)} + \Delta^2_{X(m-k-1)}] + \frac{1}{m^2 r}\sum_{i=k+1}^{m-k}\Delta^2_{X(i)}}{\overline{X}^2} = \frac{RV(\bar{x}_{\mathrm{LRSS}})}{\overline{X}^2}$$

$$C(\text{LRSS}) = \frac{\rho\sqrt{V(\bar{x}_{\text{LRSS}})V(\bar{y}_{\text{LRSS}})}}{\bar{X}^2}$$

Therefore, as $E(\bar{y}_{R(\text{LRSS})}) \cong \mu + \bar{X}B(y(\text{LRSS}))$ we have that $\bar{y}_{R(\text{LRSS})}$ is approximatley unbiased whenever the sample size $n = \text{nr} \to \infty$. Using the same-Taylor's development

$$V(\bar{y}_{R(\text{LRSS})}) = V(\bar{y}_{(\text{LRSS})}) + R^2 V(\bar{x}_{(\text{LRSS})}) - 2\rho R\sqrt{V(\bar{y}_{(\text{LRSS})})V(\bar{x}_{(\text{LRSS})})}$$

When non response are present we may impute the values of Y in the non respondents by

$$Y_{R(i)} = \bar{y}_1 \frac{r(i)X_{(i)}}{\bar{x}_1}$$

taking for $z = x$, y, $n = \text{mr}$

$$\bar{z}_1 = \frac{\sum_{i=1}^{k}\sum_{j=1}^{r} Z_{i(k+1)j}\alpha(i,j) + \sum_{i=k+1}^{m-k}\sum_{j=1}^{r} Z_{i(i)j}\alpha(i,j) + \sum_{i=m-k+1}^{m}\sum_{j=1}^{r} Z_{i(m-k)j}\alpha(i,j)}{\sum_{i=1}^{m}\sum_{j=1}^{r}\alpha(i,j)}$$

$$r(i) = \sum_{j=1}^{r}\alpha(i,j), n_1 = \sum_{i=1}^{m} r(i), n_2 = n - n_1$$

Its conditional expectation and variance are

$$E(\bar{z}_1) = \frac{k[r(k+1)\mu_{(k+1)} + r(m-k)\mu_{(m-k)}] + \sum_{i=k+1}^{m-k} r(i)\mu_{(i)}}{n_1}$$

$$V(\bar{z}_1) = \frac{k(r(k+1)\sigma_{(k+1)}^2 + r(m-k)\sigma_{(k+1)}^2] + \sum_{i=k+1}^{m-k} r(i)\sigma_{(i)}^2}{n_1^2} = \frac{\sigma_{z(1)}^2}{n_1^2}$$

We have obtained basic results for proving the following proposition.

Proposition 4.14 Take the RSS alternative to the estimator

$$\bar{y}_{\text{LRSS}(R)} = \bar{y}_1 \left[\frac{n_1\bar{x}_1 + n_2\bar{X}}{n\bar{x}_1}\right]$$

Converges to the population mean and its error is

$$E\left((\bar{y}_{\text{LRSS}(R)} - \mu)^2\right) \cong E * \left(\varepsilon_{\theta(\text{LRSS1})} - \frac{v\mu\varepsilon_{\xi(\text{LRSS}\varnothing)}\varepsilon_{\theta(\text{LRSS}\varnothing)}}{v_{\varnothing}\Xi}\right)$$

$$= \frac{1}{\vartheta_1}\left(\frac{\sigma^2}{\text{mr}} + \frac{k}{m^2 r}[\Delta_{(k+1)}^2 + \Delta_{(m-k-1)}^2] + \frac{1}{m^2 r}\sum_{i=k+1}^{m-k}\Delta_{(i)}^2\right)$$

$$- 2 * \vartheta_{\varnothing}\epsilon(v/v_{\varnothing})\rho\sigma_{\xi(\varnothing)}\sigma_{\theta(\varnothing)}$$

Proof Using the previous results note that the unconditional expectations of the deviations are

$$E\big(\varepsilon_{x(\mathrm{LRSS2})}\big) = E((\bar{x}_2 - \bar{X})) \cong \frac{\mathrm{kr}^*(1|k)\Delta_{X(k+1)} + \sum_{i=k+1}^{m-k} r^*(2|k)\Delta_{X(i)} + \mathrm{kr}^*(3|k)\Delta_{X(m-k)}}{n_2} = \frac{\bar{\varepsilon}(2,x)}{n_2}$$

$$E\big(\varepsilon_{y(\mathrm{LRSS})}\big) = E((\bar{y}_1 - \mu)) \cong \frac{\mathrm{kr}(1|k)\Delta_{(k+1)} + \sum_{i=k+1}^{m-k} r(2|k)\Delta_{(i)} + \mathrm{kr}(3|k)\Delta_{(m-k)}}{n_1} = \frac{\bar{\varepsilon}(1,y)}{n_1}$$

$$E\big(\varepsilon_{x(\mathrm{LRSS1})}\big) = E((\bar{x}_1 - \bar{X})) \cong \frac{\mathrm{kr}(1|k)\Delta_{X(k+1)} + \sum_{i=k+1}^{m-k} r(2|k)\Delta_{X(i)} + \mathrm{kr}(3|k)\Delta_{X(m-k)}}{n_1} = \frac{\bar{\varepsilon}(1,x)}{n_1}$$

Developing the Taylor Series and retaining the terms or order $O\,(h^{-2})$ and after some algebraic work we obtain that

$$\mathrm{EE}\big(\bar{y}_{\mathrm{LRSS}(R)}\big) \cong \mathrm{EE}\big(\varepsilon_{y(\mathrm{LRSS})}\big) - \mathrm{REE}\big(n_2\varepsilon_{x(\mathrm{LRSS1})}\big) - \frac{1}{n\bar{X}}\Big(\mathrm{EE}\big(n_2\varepsilon_{y(\mathrm{LRSS})}\varepsilon_{x(\mathrm{LRSS1})}\big) - \Big(\mathrm{REE}\big(n_2\varepsilon_{x(\mathrm{LRSS1})}^2\big)\Big)\Big)$$

$$= \bar{\varepsilon}(1,y)E\big(n_1^{-1}\big) - \mathrm{R}\bar{\varepsilon}(1,x)E\Big(\frac{n_2}{n_1}\Big) - E(n_2/n_1)\rho\sigma_{x_{(1)}}\sigma_{y(1)}$$

Note that they are random variables because they depend of the number of responses. We denote

$$E\big(n_1^{-1}\big) = \vartheta_1^{-1},\, E\Big(\frac{n_2}{n_1}\Big) = \vartheta_{12}$$

The approximate variance is obtained developing the Taylor Series. The result is

$$E\Big(\big(\bar{y}_{\mathrm{LRSS}(R)} - \mu\big)^2\Big) \cong E * \left(\varepsilon_{\theta(\mathrm{LRSS1})}\big) - \frac{\nu\mu\varepsilon_{\xi(\mathrm{LRSS1})}\varepsilon_{\theta(\mathrm{LRSS1})}}{\nu_\varnothing \Xi}\right)$$

$$= \frac{1}{\vartheta_1}\Big(\frac{\sigma^2}{\mathrm{mr}} + \frac{k}{m^2 r}[\Delta_{(k+1)}^2 + \Delta_{(m-k-1)}^2] + \frac{1}{m^2 r}\sum_{i=k+1}^{m-k}\Delta_{(i)}^2\Big)$$

$$- 2 * \vartheta_\varnothing \epsilon(\nu/\nu_\varnothing)\rho\sigma_{\xi_{(\varnothing)}}\sigma_{\theta(\varnothing)}$$

References

Al-Nasser, D. A. (2007): L-ranked set sampling: A generalization procedure for robust visual sampling. *Communications in Statistics: Simulation and Computation, 6*, 33–43.

Al-Omari, A. I., & Jaber, K. (2008). Percentile double ranked set sampling. *Journal of Mathematics and Statistics, 4*, 60–64.

Al-Omari, A. I., JABER, K., & Al-Omari, A. (2008). Modified ratio-type estimators of the mean using extreme ranked set sampling. *Journal of Mathematics and Statistics, 4*, 150–155.

Al-Omari, A. I., Jemain, A. A., & Ibrahim, K. (2009). New ratio estimators of the mean using simple random sampling and ranked set sampling methods. *Revista Investigación Operacional, 30*, 97–108.

Bai, Z. D., & Chen, Z. (2003). On the theory of ranked set sampling and its ramifications. *Journal of Statistical Planning and Inference, 109*, 81–99.

Bouza-Herrera C. N. (2012). Estimation of the population mean under l ranked set sampling with missing observations, aproved for publication in. *International Journal of Statistics and Probability.* doi10.1155/2012/214959

Bouza, C. N., & Al-Omari, A. I. (2011a). Ranked set estimation with imputation of the missing observations: the median estimator. *Revista Investigación Operacional, 2*, 30–37.

Bouza, C. N., & Al-Omari, A. I. (2011b). Ratio imputation of missing data in ranked set sampling. Submitted to statistics, gsta-2011-0026.r2.

Bouza, C. N., & Al-Omari, A. I. (2013). Imputation methods of missing data for estimating the population mean using simple random sampling with known correlation coefficient. Accepted by Quality and Quantity, 47, 353–365. doi 10.1007/s11135-011-9522-1.

Bouza, C. N., & Al-Omari, A. I. (2011c). Estimating the population mean in the case of missing data using simple random sampling. To be published in statistics, doi10.1080/02331888. 2010.505654.

Bouza, C. N. (2008a). Estimation of the population mean with missing observations using product type estimators. *Revista Investigación Operacional, 29*, 207–223.

Chang, H. J., & Huang, K. (2008). Ratio estimation in survey sampling when some observations are missing. *International Journal of Information and Management Sciences, 12*, 1–9.

Chang, H. J., & Huang, K. (2000b). On estimation of ratio of populatoin means in survey sampling when some observations are missing. *Journal of Information & Optimization Sciences, 21*, 429–436.

Chen, Z., Bai, Z., & Sinha, B. K. (2004). *Ranked set sampling: theory and applications.* Lectures notes in statistics, p. 176. New York: Springer.

Jemain, A. A., & Al-Omari, A. I. (2006). Multistage median ranked set samples for estimating the population mean. *Pakistan Journal of Statistics, 22*, 195–207.

Kadilar, C., & Cingi, H. (2008). Estimators for the population mean in the case of missing data. *Communication in Statistics: Theory and Methods, 37*, 2226–2236.

Liu, L., TUA, Y., LIB, Y., & ZOU, G. (2006). Imputation for missing data and variance estimation when auxiliary information is incomplete. *Model Assisted Statistics and Applications, 1*, 83–94.

Mutlak, H. A. (1997). Median ranked set sampling. *Journal of Applied Statistical Sciences, 6*, 245–255.

Muttlak, H. A. (2003). Investigating the use of quartile ranked set samples for estimating the population mean. *Journal of Applied Mathematics and Computation, 146*, 437–443.

Young-Jae, M. (2005). Monotonicity conditions and inequality imputation for sample and non-response problems. *Econometric Reviews, 24*, 175–194.

Rubin, D. B. (1976). Inference and missing data. *Biometrika, 63*, 581–582.

Rueda, M., & González, S. (2004). Missing data and auxiliary information in surveys. *Computational Statistics, 10*, 559–567.

Rueda, M., Martínez, S., Martínez, H., & Arcos, A. (2006). Mean estimation with calibration techniques in presence of missing data. *Computational Statistics and Data Analysis, 50*, 3263–3277.

Samawi, H. M., & Muttlak, H. A. (1996). Estimation of ratio using rank set sampling. *Biometrical Journal, 36*, 753–764.

Singh, S., & Deo, B. (2003). Imputation by power transformation. *Statistical Papers, 44*, 555–579.

Singh, S., & Horn, S. (2000). Compromised imputation in survey sampling. *Metrika, 51*, 267–276.

Takahasi, K., & Wakimoto, K. (1968). On unbiased estimates of population mean based on the sample stratified by means of ordering. Annals of the Institute of Statistical Mathematics, *20*, 1–31.

Toutenburg, H., Srivastava, V. K., & SHALABH, V. (2008). Amputation versus imputation of missing values through ratio method in sample surveys. *Statistical Papers, 49*, 237–247.

Tsukerman, E. V. (2004). Optimal linear estimation of missing observations (in Russian). Studies in information science. *Kazan. Lzd. Otechetsvo, 2*, 77–96.

Zou, U., Feng, S., & Qin, H. (2002). Sample rotation with missing data. *Science in China Series A, 45*, 42–63.

Chapter 5
Some Numerical Studies of the Behavior of RSS

Abstract The superiority of Ranked Set Sampling (RSS) models is measured by the comparison of the Mean Square Errors of the models with respect to their alternatives. The expressions support general evaluations of the gains in accuracy but their values depend on the underlying distribution or the characteristics of the studied population. We present some numerical studies for illustrating the behavior of RSS strategies.

Keywords Non-responses · Imputation · Randomized responses · Monte carlo simulation

> *Numbers speak all the languages.*
> Cuban Version of a Congo Proverb

5.1 Introduction

The selection of a certain RSS model is related to the gain in accuracy due to its use. This accuracy usually is measured by the difference between the mean squared error (MSE) of a RSS estimator and alternative ones. Sometimes the evaluation is more informative when we use a relative precision measure, as the ratio of the MSE's, a measure of efficiency, or the ratio of the difference between of the alternative's MSE's and the RSS MSE, a measure of the relative gain in precision. In some cases there is not a clear gain in accuracy and it is needed to analyze the behavior of the method through numerical experimentations.

We will present some numerical experimentations developed with the aims of fixing the behavior of some RSS strategies through real life data and/or by developing Monte Carlo experiments. The behavior is measured by some relative precision measure or by evaluating the mean difference between the true values of the parameter and the estimations, computed from the results obtained in the

C. N. Bouza-Herrera, *Handling Missing Data in Ranked Set Sampling*,
SpringerBriefs in Statistics, DOI: 10.1007/978-3-642-39899-5_5,
© The Author(s) 2013

experiments. Usually a relative measure is considered. Bootstrap methodology, Efron (1979), Babu and Singh (1983), Parr (1983), is usually used for deriving inferences. Some particular procedures are developed and used in the simulations. The experiments, to be presented, were conducted in our personal studies of the models.

We will use the following data bases repeatedly:

B1. Sells in supermarkets, Castro (2000). They were obtained from the study of two supermarkets developed in Xalapa, Mexico.
B2. Infestation. The data used by Bouza and Schubert (Bouza Herrera and Schubert 2003) on infestation levels in sugar cane plantations were used. Y = number of adult insects, X = number of eggs.
B3. Diminish in the area affected by psoriasis. The data were obtained in a research reported by Viada et. al. (2004). Y = affected area in moment 2, X = initial area.
B4. Blood Analysis, Castro (2000). $Y =$ contents of hemoglobin, $X =$ level of leucocytes, developed in Veracruz, Mexico in 1998.

5.2 Studies of Some Estimators in RSS

5.2.1 Antecedents

Chapter 2 has presented some popular RSS estimators. They were characterized theoretically. In this section we present some numerical studies developed for obtaining more insight into the behavior of the estimators.

A series of real life data bases are used in the studies. The usual procedure was to select samples form the data base and compare the estimators, computing the mean absolute deviation (AD) of the estimates with respect tot the true parameter. Some studies used a relative measure defined by dividing AD by the population parameter.

The behavior for certain distribution functions is analyzed in some cases.

Each section will present the study of the estimators.

5.2.2 Analysis of a Monte Carlo Experiment of the Behavior of the Estimator of the Difference of Means

We will analyze the accuracy of the proposed RSS sampling strategies for estimating the difference of means. See Bouza (2001b, 2002b). The data used were obtained from a national inquiry developed for determining the effect of *AcM murino of isotope IgG2a*. It was developed by Centro de Inmunología Molecular of Cuba the researchers aimed to estimate the diminish of the area affected by psoriasis. A sample of 200 patients was selected and a longitudinal survey was developed, the patients were evaluated in 13 occasions, see Viada et al. (2004) for details. The index called PASI (Psoriasis Severity Index) is, see Laupracis et al. (1988), was determined in each visit. We considered:

X = Value of the index at the first visit, Y = value of the index at the end of the treatment.

The set of measurements of PASI constituted an artificial population of the data base B3. It was partitioned using the non-responses at the second (U_2) and third visit (U_3). We selected a sample from s and the subsamples were determined by classifying a selected patient in U_1 if he/she assisted to the evaluation in occasions 1, 2 and 3, in U_2 if failed the second visit and in U_3 if failed the third one. The last evaluation was made for all the patients.

One hundred samples were generated and were considered as sample fractions 0.10, 0.20 and 0.50 using SRSWR and RSS. D was computed and estimated using d_{srs} and d_{rss}:

$$G_b = \sum_{t=1}^{100} \frac{|d_b - D|_t}{100D} \quad b = \text{srs, rss}$$

was used for measuring the behavior of the alternative estimators.

The results appear in Table 5.1 for $K_j = K = 2, j = 2, 3$. They sustain that RSS provided more accurate estimations than SRSWR were expected. These results give an idea of how large the gains can be. They are increased with the increase in the sample fractions. A similar result is expected for other sets of values of the sub-sampling fractions.

5.2.3 Numerical Study of Ratio Type Estimators

Some relevant papers in RSS ratio estimation are Samawi and Muttlak (1996), Al-Omari et al. (2008, 2009) and Bouza (2001a). They as well as some extensions of them are analyzed. Some data-bases were used for computing the sampling error for each estimator for RSS and SRSWR. The relative accuracy was measured by

$$RP = MSE(rss)/MSE(srs)$$

It was computed for each alternative. The results are given in the Table 5.2 considering $r = 5$ and $m = 4$. The results suggest that it is better to use in all the cases except for θ_6 y θ_7 in the study of blood. The distribution was a Gaussian.

Table 5.1 Relative mean accuracy in aercent

Sample fraction	100 G_{srs}	100 G_{rss}
0.10	13.12	4.45
0.20	09.03	2.24
0.50	08.17	1.95

Table 5.2 Relative accuracy of RSS versus SRSWR

Estimator	Supermarkets	Infestation	Área affected	Study of the blood
Classic	0.56	0.66	0.60	0.89
Singh-Taylor	0.35	0.55	0.59	0.88
θ_1	0.84	0.81	0.68	0.95
θ_2	0.66	0.73	0.61	0.92
θ_3	0.92	0.83	0.72	0.77
θ_4	0.97	0.72	0.61	0.85
θ_5	0.98	0.84	0.60	0.98
θ_6	0.89	0.87	0.55	1.07
θ_7	0.80	0.68	0.64	1.09
θ_8	0.84	0.75	0.66	0.97
θ_9	0.81	0.68	0.62	0.91
θ_{10}	0.79	0.77	0.7	0.91

The largest gain was obtained by the estimator of Singh-Taylor followed by the classic ratio estimator.

We analyzed also the behavior of the estimators generating the Gaussian case: $Y \sim > (N(0,1),\ X \sim > N(1,1))$. Using a normal standard for both variables is unnatural as we will have a un-definition of the ratio of the means. We considered that Y and X had the same distribution: the exponential case $Exp(1)$ and the *Uniform* $U(0,1)$. The moments of the involved order statistics were calculated using a Taylor Series approximation. The joint distribution were generated using the following values of the correlation coefficient $\rho \in \{-0.9, -0.5, -0.1, 0.1, 0.5, 0.9\}$.

The estimators were compared. See the corresponding tables.

The results in Table 5.3 suggest that a larger gain in accuracy is obtained for the exponential with negative values of ρ.

The results for the estimator of Singh and Taylor (2003) in Table 5.4 fix that if the expectation is cero ρ is unimportant in the study of the accuracy. When ρ is negative RSS is the best strategy. Again the best results for RSS are obtained for the $E(1)$.

Table 5.3 Relative accuracy of RSS versus srs for the classic ratio estimator

Distribution	$\rho = -0.9$	$\rho = -0.5$	$\rho = -0.1$	$\rho = 0.1$	$\rho = 0.5$	$\rho = 0.9$
Gaussian	0.33	0.46	0.52	0.67	0.71	0.82
$E(1)$	0.21	0.30	0.34	0.39	0.43	0.48
$U(0,1)$	0.46	0.49	0.51	0.54	0.55	0.59

Table 5.4 Relative accuracy of RSS versus srs for the estimator of: singh and taylor

Distribution	$\rho = -0.9$	$\rho = -0.5$	$\rho = -0.1$	$\rho = 0.1$	$\rho = 0.5$	$\rho = 0.9$
Gaussian	0.43	0.43	0.43	0.43	0.43	0.43
$E(1)$	0.28	0.23	0.24	0.18	0.13	0.11
$U(0,1)$	0.74	0.72	0.69	0.62	0.68	0.72

Table 5.5 Relative accuracy of RSS versus SRS for the estimators of Kadilar and Cingi

Distribution	$\rho = -0.9$	$\rho = -0.5$	$\rho = -0.1$	$\rho = 0.1$	$\rho = 0.5$	$\rho = 0.9$
θ_1						
Gaussian	0.53	0.45	0.40	0.40	0.45	0.53
$E(1)$	0.41	0.38	0.27	0.27	0.38	0.41
$U(0,1)$	0.69	0.55	0.49	0.49	0.55	0.69
θ_2						
Gaussian	0.51	0.46	0.38	0.38	0.46	0.51
$E(1)$	0.43	0.39	0.24	0.24	0.39	0.43
$U(0,1)$	0.68	0.57	0.51	0.51	0.57	0.68
θ_3						
Gaussian	0.55	0.49	0.40	0.40	0.49	0.55
$E(1)$	0.40	0.38	0.27	0.27	0.38	0.40
$U(0,1)$	0.66	0.58	0.52	0.52	0.58	0.66
θ_4						
Gaussian	0.47	0.40	0.38	0.38	0.40	0.47
$E(1)$	0.41	0.35	0.30	0.30	0.35	0.41
$U(0,1)$	0.78	0.74	0.71	0.71	0.74	0.78
θ_5						
Gaussian	0.56	0.52	0.48	0.48	0.52	0.56
$E(1)$	0.39	0.36	0.33	0.33	0.36	0.39
$U(0,1)$	0.67	0.64	0.61	0.61	0.64	0.67
θ_6						
Gaussian	0.55	0.49	0.40	0.40	0.49	0.55
$E(1)$	0.40	0.38	0.27	0.27	0.38	0.40
$U(0,1)$	0.66	0.58	0.52	0.52	0.58	0.66
θ_7						
Gaussian	0.55	0.45	0.40	0.40	0.45	0.55
$E(1)$	0.40	0.38	0.35	0.35	0.38	0.40
$U(0,1)$	0.66	0.58	0.53	0.53	0.58	0.66
θ_8						
Gaussian	0.66	0.49	0.40	0.40	0.49	0.66
$E(1)$	0.40	0.37	0.27	0.27	0.37	0.40
$U(0,1)$	0.69	0.67	0.62	0.62	0.67	0.69
θ_9						
Gaussian	0.48	0.40	0.36	0.36	0.40	0.48
$E(1)$	0.41	0.35	0.30	0.30	0.35	0.41
$U(0,1)$	0.58	0.54	0.51	0.51	0.54	0.58
θ_{10}						
Gaussian	0.57	0.50	0.38	0.38	0.50	0.57
$E(1)$	0.51	0.35	0.30	0.30	0.35	0.51
$U(0,1)$	0.68	0.65	0.60	0.60	0.65	0.68

Table 5.5 presents the results for the estimator developed by Kandilar-Cingi. In every case RSS was the best alternative.

5.2.4 Numerical Study of Other Estimators

The measurement of the accuracy was RP = MSE (A_{rss})/MSE(srs). We consider the case m even and $r = 5$, $m = 4$.

Take the median RSS sampling (MRSS) proposed by Muttlak (1995, 1998 and 2003). The estimator and its variance are:

$$\mu_{rss[med]} = \frac{\sum_{j=1}^{m} \sum_{t=1}^{r} Y_{(j:med)t}^{*}}{mr}$$

$$V\left(\mu_{Y_{rss[med]}}\right) = \frac{\sum_{j=1}^{m} \sigma_{Y_{(j:med)}}^{2}}{m^2 r} = \frac{\sigma_Y^2}{n} - \frac{\sum_{j=1}^{m} \Delta_{Y_{(j:med)}}^{2}}{mn}$$

As the bias is

$$B\left(\mu_{rss[med]}\right) = \frac{\sum_{j=1}^{m} \mu_{Y_{(j:med)}}}{m} - \mu_Y$$

the MD is

$$MSE\left(\mu_{Y_{rss[med]}}\right) = \frac{\sigma_Y^2}{n} - \frac{\sum_{j=1}^{m} \Delta_{Y_{(j:med)}}^{2}}{mn} + \left(\frac{\sum_{j=1}^{m} \mu_{Y_{(j:med)}}}{m} - \mu_Y\right)^2$$

The extreme RSS sampling (ERSS) was developed by Samawi et al. (1996a and b), Muttlak (2001), Bhoj (1997) used the estimator

$$\mu_{Y_{rss(e)}} = \frac{\sum_{j=1}^{m} Y_{(j:e)}}{m}$$

and

$$V\left(\mu_{Y_{rss(e)}}\right) = \frac{\sigma_{Y_{(1)}}^2 + \sigma_{Y(m)}^2}{2m}$$

As

$$B\left(\mu_{Y_{rss(e)}}\right) = \frac{\mu_{Y_{(1)}} + \mu_{Y_{(m)}}}{2} - \mu_Y$$

$$MSE\left(\mu_{Y_{rss(e)}}\right) = \frac{\sigma_{Y_{(1)}}^2 + \sigma_{Y(m)}^2}{2m} + \left(\frac{\mu_{Y_{(1)}} + \mu_{Y(m)}}{2} - \mu_Y\right)^2$$

Table 5.6 Relative accuracy of the median and extreme RSS estimators versus srs

Estimator	Supermarkets	Infestation	Área affected	Study of the blood
$\mu_{rss[med]}$	2.14	1.57	1.53	1.08
$\mu_{Y_{rss(e)}}$	1.14	2.63	2.46	1.11

We instrumented the same experiment with the data bases for these estimators and obtained the results in the Table 5.6.

The results obtained sustain that these estimators are not recommendable for studying problems similar to those of the data bases. Particularly their best results are for the study of the blood, where the normality can be accepted.

5.3 Analysis of Non-response Models

5.3.1 Introduction

RSS for non responses (NR) was the subject of Chap. 3. The behavior of the non respondents depends of different external causes. Therefore the development of numerical analysis gives an idea of what is to be expected in applications. Monte Carlo experiments mimic some non response mechanisms. As in previous sections the behavior of the RSS procedures is evaluated by means of computing efficiency and/or relative precision. The basic theory appears in a series of papers, see Bouza (2002a), Kadilar and Cingi (2008), Rueda and González (2004) for example.

5.3.2 A Monte Carlo Comparison of the Accuracy for Estimating the Population Mean

The comparison was developed using two data base sets. They provided the set of values of the interest variable Y in the population: $Y_1, \ldots Y_N$. Some of the Y_j's are identified as non-respondents. They correspond to units for which the first measurement was inaccurate and a second visit was made for obtaining a correct evaluation. Hence, once a sample s was selected we were able to identify s_1 and s_2. In our notation each RSS procedure is identified with:

$$R = \text{RSS, ERSS, MRSS.}$$

The Monte Carlo experiment worked as follows:

Step 1: We select s then the sample mean of Y in s_1 is calculated and n'_2 is determined.

Step 2: We select n'_2 sub-samples from s_2 and they are ranked.

Step 3: A Bootstrap procedure selects re-samples of size n'_2 using srswr from each of the n'_2 sub-samples.

Step 4: For each $b + 1, \ldots, B$ the Bootstrap estimate of μ:

$$\bar{\bar{y}}_{(R)mb} w_1 \bar{y}_1 + w_2 \bar{y}'_{(2R)b}$$

is computed for the m-th sample using

$$\bar{\bar{y}}_{(erss)} = w_1 \bar{y}'_{2(erss)} = w_1 \bar{y}_1 + w_2 \bar{y}'_{2(erss)}$$

$$\bar{\bar{y}}_{(rss)} = \frac{n_1}{n} \bar{y}_1 + \frac{n_2}{n} \bar{y}'_{2(rss)} = w_1 \bar{y}_1 + w_2 \bar{y}'_{2(rss)}$$

correspondingly to each R.

The cycle is repeated for obtaining M samples. Then the variance is estimated and the Bootstrap confidence interval (CI) is calculated using the B obtained Bootstrap's samples. As we know the real value of μ we can compute the proportion of times that the CI contains it. R identifies the RSS estimator to be used for estimating the non-respondent's stratum means.

The Bootstrap procedure algorithm used is described as follows.

BOOTSTRAP PROCEDURE

Fix $Y = \{Y_1,\ldots, Y_N\}$, K, M and B.

While $m < M$ do

$m = 0$, $h = 0$, $\pi(R) = 0$

Select a sample $\{y_1,\ldots,y_n\}$ from Y using simple random sampling with replacement.

If y_j is a non-respondent then $y_j \in s_2, |s_2| = n_2, |\{j \in s_2\}| = n_1, n'_2 = \lfloor n_2/K \rfloor$

$$w_1 = n_1/n, \; w_2 = n_2/n$$

$$\text{Compute } \bar{y}_1 = \frac{\displaystyle\sum_{j \notin s_2} y_j}{n_1}$$

While $b < B$ do

While $h < n'_2$ do

Select a sample $s_{2h} = \{y_1,\ldots,y_{n2'}\}$ from s_2 using simple random sampling with replacement.

Rank s_{2h} and determine the ranked sample $s_2(h)$

$$h = h + 1$$

Select using srswr a Bootstrap subsample s_{2hb} from s_{2h}

$$\text{Compute} \qquad \bar{y}_{(R)b} = \frac{\displaystyle\sum_{j=1}^{n'_2} y_{(j:R)b}}{n'_2}$$

$$\bar{\bar{y}}_{(R)mb} \quad w_1 \bar{y}_1 + w_2 \bar{y}'_{(2R)b}$$

$$b = b + 1$$

Calculate

$$\overline{\overline{y}}_{(R)mB} = \frac{\sum_{b=1}^{B} \overline{\overline{y}}_{(R)mb}}{B}$$

$$s_{(R)mB} = \sqrt{\frac{\sum_{b=1}^{B} \left(\overline{\overline{y}}_{(R)mb} - \overline{\overline{y}}_{(R)mB} \right)^2}{B-1}}$$

$$I_{(R)mB} = \left(\overline{\overline{y}}_{(R)mB} - \frac{2s_{(R)mb}}{\sqrt{B}}, \overline{\lambda} + \frac{2s_{(R)mB}}{\sqrt{B}} \right)$$

$$Z_{(R)m} = \begin{cases} 1 & \text{if} \qquad \mu \in I_{(R)mB} \\ 0 & \text{otherwise} \end{cases}$$

$$\pi(R) = \pi(R) + Z_{(R)m}$$

$$M = M + 1$$

$$\pi(R) = \pi(R)/M$$

END

Note that the CI uses 2 as an approximation of the 95 % percentile.

We used $K = 2$, 5 and 10, B/n $\cong$ 0.1, 0.2 and 0.5 f = $n/N \cong$ 0.1, 0.05 and 0.01 and $M = 100$. Considering the proportions $\rho(R)$, the relative evaluation of a method's precision is measured by:

$$\rho(R) = \sum_{m=1}^{M} \left| \mu_{(R)} - \mu \right|_m / M\mu$$

where $\mu(R)$ is the estimator of the mean μ made by the corresponding RSS estimator.

Analyzing Table 5.7 we may consider that the use of RSS for sub-sampling the non-respondents, in the study of sugar cane infestation, provided the best coverage of μ. It is acceptable in any case. For $f = 0.10$ the obtained percentages of coverage are close to the nominal $\alpha = 0.05$ for any value of the sub-sampling rule parameter K. For the rest of the values of f it is not so close except when $K = 2$. The use of ERSS provided what may be considered as an acceptable coverage only for f = 0.1 and $K = 2$. The results for MRSS are not satisfactory in any case. With the increment in B the situation is very similar. Then it seems that B does not sensibly affect the behavior of the proposed estimators.

Table 5.8 presents the percentage of coverage of μ by the Bootstrap CI's computed using samples from the data providing from Hemoglobin's analysis. Again the use of RSS is the best option but MRSS has a good behavior for $f = 0.1$ and $f = 0.05$ as well as when $B/n \cong 0.5$. The increase in this parameter is generally associated with better values of $\pi(MRSS)$. These results may be generated by the fact that the percent in hemoglobin is well described by a normal distribution. The behavior of ERSS again is poor.

Table 5.7 Percent of coverage of the confidence intervals: $100\pi(R)$ for the variable $Y =$ Coefficient of infestation in sugar cane fields

$B/n \cong 0.1$									
Subsample	.RSS			ERSS			.MRSS		
Parameter	$f = 0.1$	$f = 0.05$	$f = 0.01$	$f = 0.1$	$f = 0.05$	$f = 0.01$	$f = 0.1$	$f = 0.05$	$f = 0.01$
$K = 2$	96.78	93.24	92.53	89.41	83.69	84.30	81.48	79.45	77.61
.$K = 5$	94.23	89.45	91.10	84.44	81.69	81.84	81.17	78.48	73.53
$K = 10$	94.09	89.62	91.04	84.66	80.798	81.29	81.38	77.68	71.89
$B/n \cong 0.2$									
$K = 2$	96.87	93.31	92.84	89.32	83.42	85.23	82.18	80.11	77.84
.$K = 5$	94.44	89.26	91.17	84.02	81.44	81.38	81.67	78.83	73.22
$K = 10$	94.29	89.19	90.38	84.08	80.30	81.66	81.54	77.88	71.67
$B/n \cong 0.5$									
$K = 2$	96.77	93.33	92.09	89.09	83.38	84.42	81.73	79.93	77.54
.$K = 5$	94.19	89.31	91.12	84.03	81.79	81.88	81.19	77.49	73.69
$K = 10$	94.10	89.19	91.03	84.07	80.88	81.39	81.89	77.31	71.07

Table 5.8 Percent of coverage of the confidence intervals: $100\pi(R)$ for the variable $Y =$ Hemoglobin in blood in adolescents

$B/n \cong 0.1$									
Subsample	.RSS			ERSS			.MRSS		
Parameter	$f = 0.1$	$f = 0.05$	$f = 0.01$	$f = 0.1$	$f = 0.05$	$f = 0.01$	$f = 0.1$	$f = 0.05$	$f = 0.01$
$K = 2$	95.45	93.21	90.02	89.39	83.71	84.26	94.25	92.00	89.42
.$K = 5$	94.72	91.37	93.63	84.35	81.74	81.81	93.58	91.03	87.44
$K = 10$	94.33	91.11	90.37	84.67	80.8	81.33	92.86	94.51	85.03
$B/n \cong 0.2$									
$K = 2$	93.42	92.88	92.92	89.33	83.39	85.20	97.49	95.14	92.00
.$K = 5$	92.37	90.04	90.61	84.02	81.36	81.37	91.11	93.67	91.69
$K = 10$	92.21	94.32	93.00	84.13	80.31	81.74	92.30	91.38	88.39
$B/n \cong 0.5$									
$K = 2$	95.40	90.01	90.58	89.08	83.44	84.40	94.84	92.67	92.86
.$K = 5$	95.28	94.39	93.14	84.01	81.82	81.92	94.32	89.62	91.59
$K = 10$	94.69	94.03	90.30	84.13	80.90	81.39	95.80	90.54	91.71

A look to Table 5.9 suggests that for RSS the increment of f and a disminish in K have a significant influence in obtaining small values of $\rho(RSS)$. It seems that the levels of f and K have not a significant influence in $\rho(RSS)$. A similar comment may be made on the behavior of ERSS. This procedure is considerably more inaccurate than RSS. $\rho(MRSS)$ is always smaller than $\rho(ERSS)$ for $f = 0.1$ it performs better than RSS for $K = 2$.

The results given in Table 5.10 suggest that for RSS the increment of K determines larger value of $\rho(RSS)$. It seems that the levels of f have not a significant influence in $\rho(RSS)$. ERSS has a worse behavior compared with the other procedures. Its accuracy is seriously affected by the increments in K and f. MRSS has a better behavior than RSS which is not seriously affected by changes

Table 5.9 Values of $\rho(R)$ for the variable $Y =$ Coefficient of infestation in sugar cane fields

Subsample	.RSS			ERSS			.MRSS		
Parameter	$f = 0.1$	$f = 0.05$	$f = 0.01$	$f = 0.1$	$f = 0.05$	$f = 0.01$	$f = 0.1$	$f = 0.05$	$f = 0.01$
$K = 2$	0.431	0.477	0.52	0.988	0.962	0.943	0.420	0.421	0.441
.$K = 5$	0.513	0.503	0.56	0.986	0.923	0.872	0.427	0.573	0.594
$K = 10$	0.560	0.534	0.56	0.967	0.918	0.977	0.488	0.559	0.592

Table 5.10 Values of $\rho(R)$ for the variable $Y =$ Hemoglobin in blood in adolescents

Subsample	.RSS			ERSS			.MRSS		
Parameter	$f = 0.1$	$f = 0.05$	$f = 0.01$	$f = 0.1$	$f = 0.05$	$f = 0.01$	$f = 0.1$	$f = 0.05$	$f = 0.01$
$K = 2$	0.274	0.222	0.288	0.667	0.622	0.629	0.214	0.212	0.256
.$K = 5$	0.372	0.289	0.338	0.804	0.724	0.727	0.213	0.237	0.214
$K = 10$	0.420	0.313	0.311	0.942	0.842	0.852	0.203	0.219	0.263

in any of the parameters. Again the possible normality of the involved variable should be having a determinant influence in the behavior of the accuracy of MRSS.

5.3.3 Estimation of the Difference of Means: Analysis of a Monte Carlo Experiment

We will analyze the accuracy of the proposals using the same data as in 5.2: the effect of *AcM murino of isotope IgG2a.* in diminishing the area affected by psoriasis by means of PASI (Psoriasis Severity Index) is).

Experiment 1:

The set of measurements of PASI constituted an artificial population. It was partitioned using the non-responses at the second (U_2) and third visit. (U_3). We selected a sample from s and the subsamples were determined by classifying a selected patient in U_1 if he/she assisted to the evaluation in occasions 1, 2 and 3, in U_2 if failed the second visit and in U_3 if failed the third one. The last evaluation was made for all the patients.

100 samples were generated and with sample fractions of 0.10, 0.20 and 0.50 using SRSWR and RSS. D was computed and estimated using d_{srs} and d_{rss}. The relative accuracy:

$$G_b = \sum_{t=1}^{100} \frac{|d_b - D|_t}{100D} \qquad b = \mathrm{srs}, \mathrm{rss} \text{ was used for measuring the behavior of the}$$

alternative estimators.

The results appear in Table 5.11 for $K_j = K = 2$, j = 2, 3. They sustain that RSS provided more accurate estimations than srs were expected. These results give an idea of how large the gains are. They are increased with the increase in the

Table 5.11 Relative mean accuracy in percent

Sample fraction	$100G_{\mathrm{srs}}$	$100G_{\mathrm{rss}}$
0.10	13.12	4.45
0.20	9.03	2.24
0.50	8.17	1.95

sample fractions. A similar result is expected for other sets of values of the sub-sampling fractions.

Experiment 2:

We used the data base sets of 200 the PASI of 200 patients, it is normal variable, and the percent of infestation of a pest in 1500 measurements made in sugar cane fields, which is has a skewed distribution. They provided the set of values of the interest variable Y in the population: $Y_1,\ldots Y_N$. Some of the Y_j's are identified as non-respondents. They correspond to units for which the first measurement was inaccurate or and a second visit was made for obtaining a correct evaluation. Hence, once a sample s was selected we were able to identify s_1 and s_2. In our notation each RSS procedure is identified with $R = $ RSS, ERSS, MRSS.

The Monte Carlo experiment worked as follows:

Step 1:   We select s then the sample mean of Y in s_1 is calculated and n'_2 is determined.
Step 2:   We select n'_2 sub-samples from s_2 and they are ranked.
Step 3:   Calculate the srswr estimator in each sample.
Step 4:   Calculate the estimator in each RSS alternative (Table 5.12).

$$\rho(R) = \sum_{m=1}^{M} \left| \mu_{(R)} - \mu \right|_m / M\mu$$

for the RSS estimator and for srswr

$$\rho(R) = \sum_{m=1}^{M} \sum_{t=1}^{n'(m,2)} |\mu(R) - \mu|_m / Mn'(m,2)\mu$$

where $n'(m, 2)$ is the number size of s'_2 in the generated sample m.

Analyzing Table 5.13 we may consider that the use of RSS for sub-sampling the non-respondents, in the study of sugar cane infestation, provided the best coverage of μ. It is acceptable in any case. For $f = 0.10$ the obtained percentages of coverage are close to the nominal $\alpha = 0.05$ for any value of the sub-sampling rule parameter K. For the rest of the values of f it is not so close except when $K = 2$. The use of eRSS provided what may be considered as an acceptable coverage only for $f = 0.1$ and $K = 2$. The results for MRSS are not satisfactory in any case. With the increment in B the situation is very similar. Then it seems that B does not sensibly affect the behavior of the proposed estimators.

Table 5.12 Values of $\rho(R)$ for the variable Y = PASI

K	SRSWR			RSS			ERSS			MRSS		
	$f = 0.1$	$f = 0.05$	$f = 0.01$	$f = 0.1$	$f = 0.05$	$f = 0.01$	$f = 0.1$	$f = 0.05$	$f = 0.01$	$f = 0.1$	$f = 0.05$	$f = 0.01$
2	1.50	1.54	1.68	1.09	1.11	1.20	1.16	1.22	1.26	1.15	1.15	1.24
5	1.22	1.31	1.32	1.04	1.09	1.15	1.12	1.17	1.20	1.09	1.21	1.12
10	0.77	1.08	1.12	0.64	0.92	1.02	1.09	1.10	1.13	0.99	1.11	1.18

Table 5.13 Percent of coverage of the confidence intervals: $100\pi(R)$ for the variable Y = Coefficient of infestation in sugar cane fields

$B/n \cong 0.1$									
Subsample	.RSS			ERSS			.MRSS		
Parameter	$f = 0.1$	$f = 0.05$	$f = 0.01$	$f = 0.1$	$f = 0.05$	$f = 0.01$	$f = 0.1$	$f = 0.05$	$f = 0.01$
$K = 2$	96.81	93.19	92.45	89.44	83.67	84.32	81.47	79.54	77.60
$.K = 5$	94.19	89.48	91.03	84.38	81.69	81.89	81.23	78.49	73.48
$K = 10$	94.14	89.56	91.02	84.68	80.77	81.27	81.38	77.70	71.89
$B/n \cong 0.2$									
$K = 2$	96.88	93.27	92.83	89.33	83.38	85.20	82.22	80.07	77.83
$.K = 5$	94.43	89.33	91.19	84.02	81.39	81.43	81.71	78.79	73.21
$K = 10$	94.31	89.24	90.37	84.14	80.31	81.73	81.53	77.89	71.66
$B/n \cong 0.5$									
$K = 2$	96.83	93.32	92.11	89.09	83.42	84.38	81.69	79.89	77.48
$.K = 5$	94.17	89.29	91.14	84.03	81.88	81.86	81.22	77.49	73.69
$K = 10$	94.11	89.21	91.02	84.08	80.89	81.39	81.89	77.32	71.23

Table 5.14 presents the percentage of coverage of μ by the Bootstrap CI's computed using samples from the data providing from Hemoglobin's analysis. Again the use of RSS is the best option but MRSS has a good behavior for $f = 0.1$ and $f = 0.05$ as well as when $B/n \cong 0.5$. The increase in this parameter is generally associated with better values of π(MRSS). These results may be generated by the fact that the percent in hemoglobin is well described by a normal distribution. The behavior of ERSS again is poor.

A look to Table 5.15 suggests that for RSS the increment of f and a diminishing in K have a significant influence in obtaining small values of ρ(RSS). It seems that the levels of f and K have not a significant influence in ρ(RSS). A similar comment may be made on the behavior of ERSS. This procedure is considerably more

Table 5.14 Percent of coverage of the confidence intervals: $100\pi(R)$ for the variable Y = Hemoglobin in blood in adolescents

$B/n \cong 0.1$									
Subsample	.RSS			ERSS			.MRSS		
Parameter	$f = 0.1$	$f = 0.05$	$f = 0.01$	$f = 0.1$	$f = 0.05$	$f = 0.01$	$f = 0.1$	$f = 0.05$	$f = 0.01$
$K = 2$	95.53	93.23	90.04	89.38	83.74	84.33	94.314	92.02	89.37
$.K = 5$	94.66	91.40	93.60	84.42	81.73	81.82	93.6	91.04	87.41
$K = 10$	94.32	91.12	90.36	84.70	80.79	81.34	92.90	94.48	85.00
	0								
$B/n \cong 0.2$									
$K = 2$	93.40	92.88	92.89	89.31	83.42	85.24	97.53	95.11	92.03
$.K = 5$	92.41	90.03	90.64	84.04	81.38	81.40	91.13	93.73	91.71
$K = 10$	92.21	94.34	93.01	84.12	80.32	81.74	92.28	91.40	88.37
$B/n \cong 0.5$									
$K = 2$	95.37	90.02	90.58	89.07	83.39	84.40	94.78	92.72	92.9
$.K = 5$	95.28	94.38	93.12	84.02	81.84	81.88	94.33	89.63	91.61
$K = 10$	94.70	94.04	90.30	84.11	80.92	81.39	95.84	90.45	91.69

Table 5.15 Values of $\rho(R)$ for the variable $Y =$ Coefficient of infestation in sugar cane fields

Subsample	.RSS			ERSS			.MRSS		
Parameter	$f = 0.1$	$f = 0.05$	$f = 0.01$	$f = 0.1$	$f = 0.05$	$f = 0.01$	$f = 0.1$	$f = 0.05$	$f = 0.01$
$K = 2$	0.426	0.480	0.519	0.993	0.962	0.944	0.421	0.418	0.439
.$K = 5$	0.509	0.503	0.558	0.991	0.919	0.866	0.433	0.569	0.586
$K = 10$	0.563	0.528	0.562	0.968	0.920	0.979	0.489	0.562	0.577

Table 5.16 Values of $\rho(R)$ for the variable $Y =$ Hemoglobin in blood in adolescents

Subsample	.RSS			ERSS			.MRSS		
Parameter	$f = 0.1$	$f = 0.05$	$f = 0.01$	$f = 0.1$	$f = 0.05$	$f = 0.01$	$f = 0.1$	$f = 0.05$	$f = 0.01$
$K = 2$	0.272	0.223	0.293	0.673	0.623	0.633	0.214	0.208	0.264
.$K = 5$	0.374	0.286	0.344	0.802	0.719	0.734	0.212	0.237	0.214
$K = 10$	0.417	0.306	0.307	0.938	0.840	0.849	0.204	0.218	0.255

inaccurate than RSS. ρ(mRSS) is always smaller than ρ(eRSS) for $f = 0.1$ it performs better than RSS for $K = 2$.

The results given in Table 5.16 suggest that for RSS the increment of K determines larger value of ρ(RSS). It seems that the levels of f have not a significant influence in ρ(RSS). ERSS has a worse behavior compared with the other procedures. Its accuracy is seriously affected by the increments in K and f. MRSS has a better behavior than RSS which is not seriously affected by changes in any of the parameters. Again the possible normality of the involved variable should be having a determinant influence in the behavior of the accuracy of mRSS.

5.4   Numerical Studies of Imputation Methods

5.4.1   Some General Remarks

Chapter 4 was devoted to the study of some imputation procedures and RSS. They used some additional information for avoiding to sub sample among the non respondents. The methods are important by themselves as RSS provides additional information through the ranking. Some key references are Liu et al. (2006), Little and Rubin (1987), Singh and Deo (2003). The kernel of imputations is whether non responses are generated by a random mechanism or not. The generated $MSE's$ error formulas are rather complicated for explaining the increase in the precision due to the use of RSS.

It makes sense to evaluate the methods by comparing the imputed estimate with the true parameter. Therefore the experiments presented below deal generally with evaluating the relative MD.

5.4.2 The Median Estimator

The error of the missing observation estimator is

$$\varepsilon(\mu*_{Y(\text{rss})}) \approx 1/2[\mu^2_{(n/2)}rQ(1) + \mu^2_{(1+n/2)}rQ(1)] + s^2_{(n/2)} + s^2_{(1+n/2)}]/2nP(1)$$

We develop a numerical comparison using this measure.

We will consider the efficiency of the proposals with respect to the corresponding full response models. 1,000 samples of size 100 and a 10 % of non-responses were generated with median friendly distributions. Defining $e(I, i)$ and $e(i)$ as the estimator using the imputation and the full response one. The efficiency measure used was

$$\xi e((I, i)) = \sum |e(I, i) - \mu_Y|_h / \sum |e(I, i) - \mu_Y|_h$$

The same distribution was used for describing the behaviour of X and Y.

The results are given in Table 5.17. Note that the imputation works very well for the normal and the Laplace distributions. For the uniform it doubles the error. The ratio-product estimator.

To study the properties of imputation based estimator, are often considered through the consideration of a super population model, the sampling mechanism generating the sample, the variable response mechanism and the imputation mechanism. The properties of the variance estimators rely, among others, on the assumption.

C.1: the complete-sample point estimator $\theta*_n$ satisfies $E(\theta*_n) = \theta + O(n^{-1})$:

It is not accomplished neither by $\bar{y}_{\text{IC}} = \frac{n_1\bar{y}_1 + n_2\bar{y}*_{2p}}{n}$ nor by $\bar{y}_{\text{IS}} = \frac{n_1\bar{y}_1 + n_2\bar{y}**_{2p}}{n}$, see Chap. 4.

Hence to develop an estimator of the variances of the proposed estimators must cope with this disadvantage. The posed statistical problem is to obtain an interval $I(\theta)$ of minimum volume for a fixed probability π. Usually the methods are supported by a particular Central Limit Theorem that must establish that when $m \to \infty$

$$\text{Prob}\,(\theta) \in \{I^*(\theta) = (\theta(F_m) - z_{1-\alpha/2}\sigma_m(\theta^*_m), (\theta(F_m) + z_{1-\alpha/2}\sigma_m(\theta(F_m)))\} \geq \pi$$

$\theta(F_m)$ is the estimator (predictor) of the parameter, $z_{1-\alpha/2}$ is the percentile of the Standard Normal and $\sigma_m(\theta(F_m))$ is the standard deviation estimator of $\sigma(\theta(F))$. The robustness of $\theta(F_m)$ and $\sigma_m(\theta(F_m))$ play a key role in the validity that π be close to the coverage probability.

The Bootstrap, introduced by Efron (1979), is a powerful tool for nonparametric estimation of sampling distributions and standard errors. It may be described as follows. Let $Z = (Z_1; Z_2; : : :; Z_m)$ be a random sample from an unknown distribution F, and let $T_m = T_m(Z; F)$ be a statistic of interest. Let F_m be the empirical distribution function of the random sample. An independent random sample from F_m, Z_b, is called a Bootstrap sample. We can use the Bootstrap method for

Table 5.17 Efficiency of the developed imputation estimators versus the corresponding full response

		Uniform (0.1)		Normal (0.1)		Laplace(0.1)	
n	r	mimp	rimp	mimp	rimp	mimp	rimp
2	2	2.29	2.35	1.73	1.62	2.35	1.41
3	2	2.28	2.34	1.72	1.67	2.35	1.97
4	2	2.42	2.34	1.73	1.59	1.73	1.66
5	2	2.23	2.35	1.71	1.62	1.70	1.51
2	3	2.22	2.32	1.90	1.90	1.63	1.43
3	3	2.03	2.29	2.23	2.73	1.69	1.58
4	3	2.28	2.35	1.71	1.62	1.66	1.58
5	3	2.22	2.36	1.72	1.72	1.98	1.63
2	4	2.32	2.37	1.65	1.25	1.73	1.65
3	4	2.24	2.35	1.72	1.62	1.66	1.71
4	4	2.56	2.42	1.77	1.17	1.46	1.45
5	4	2.29	2.43	1.88	1.68	1.99	1.51
2	5	2.80	2.35	1.72	1.62	1.66	1.61
3	5	2.37	2.36	1.72	1.72	1.68	1.71
4	5	2.44	2.37	1.70	1.20	1.85	1.71
5	5	2.39	2.35	1.72	1.62	1.66	1.65

estimating the distribution of T_m through the conditional distribution of $T_{b(m)} = T_m$ $(\mathbf{Z}; F_m)$, given $Z_1; Z_2; \ldots ; Z_m$. The method works by drawing B Bootstrap samples selected by using simple random samples of size m, selected with replacement from the original sample.

The Bootstrap distribution is denoted by $F^*_{B(m)}$ and $T^*_m = T(F_{B(m)}*) = T(Z^*_1, .., Z^*_m)$ estimates $T(F_m)$. Due to the definitions, the conditional independence is supported and $\text{Prob}(Z_i* = Z_t|F_m) = 1/m$, $\forall t = 1, \ldots, m, i = 1, \ldots, m$. Each sample $s(b) \in S(BS)$, $S(BS)$ the space of the Boostrap samples, is drawn with a probability $1/m^m$, hence

$$E\big(T * \big(F*_{B(m)}\big)|F_m\big) = m^{-m} \sum_{s(b) \in S(BS)} T\big(Z*_{1, \ldots,} Z*_m\big)_b = m^{-m} \sum_{s(b) \in S(BS)} T_{B(m)}.$$

Its conditional error is $E\big(T * (F*_m) - T_m|F_m\big)^2 = m^{-m} \sum_{s(b) \in S(BS)}$ $\big(T_{B(m)} - T_m\big)^2$. It converges to σ_T^2 if $n \to \infty$. In practice we select B random samples independently from $S(BS)$ and T_{nb}, is calculated for $s(b), b = 1, \ldots, B$. The Boostrap estimator of the variance is

$$V^*_{B(m)} = (mB)^{-1} \sum_{b=1}^{B} \big(T_{B(m)} - T_m\big)^2 = \sigma^2_{B(m)}$$

It is expected, if the functional is smooth, that the limit of $\sigma^2_{B(m)}$ is the true variance of the estimator (predictor). A Central Limit Theorem supports that

Prob $(\theta) \in \{I * (\theta)$
$$= (\theta(F_m) - z_{1-\alpha/2}\sigma_{B(m)}(\theta*_m), \ (\theta(F_m) + z_{1-\alpha/2}\sigma_{B(m)}(\theta(F_m))\} \geq \pi$$

Note that the accuracy of $\theta*_m$ may be measured using its distribution function by estimating the confidence limits based on

$$L(Z_1,\ldots,Z_m) = L_m = Sup\,\{t|\,F_q(z) \geq t\}, \ U(Z_1,\ldots,Z_m) = U_m$$
$$= Inf\,\{t|\,F_\theta(z) \leq t\}$$

The interval (L_n, U_n) has random bounds and the coverage probability of θ, π is such that

$$Prob_\theta\{T(F) = \theta \in (L_m, U_m)\} \geq \pi, \text{ for any } \theta.$$

Usually $\pi = 1\text{-}\alpha$ is fixed as a value close to 1.

An alternative confidence interval, see Parr (1983) and Babu and Singh (1983) for example, is obtained by defining the parameter as the functional $\theta(F)$, $F \in \Upsilon$, and to denote the confidence interval from the relationship $Prob_F\{\theta(F) \in (L_m, U_m) = I(\theta)\,|\,F \in \Upsilon\} \geq \pi$. The Bootstrap distribution allows to calculate directly the quantiles $F*_m(t) = B^{-1}\Phi^B_{b=1}I((T_{B(m)} - T_m)m^{-1/2} \leq t)$, $t \in \Re$.

They converge, under weak regularity conditions, see Jurečkovà-Sen (1996), $\sigma^2_{B(m)} \to \sigma^2_T$ and the quantiles of $F*_m$ to those of the true distribution function of the data G, whenever, for $m \to \infty$

$$P_F\{(T(F_m) - T(F))m^{-1/2} \leq t\} \to G(t)$$

The first intervals will be called *normalized Bootstrap* (parametric) and the second ones *Bootstrap quantiles* (non parametric) confidence intervals.

We evaluate the behavior of the estimators proposed by computing the percent of samples in which the mean is included in the confidence intervals

$$I(\mu_Y)_q = \left(\widehat{\mu}_{Y\upsilon(q)} - \varepsilon_{Yp\upsilon(q)}, \widehat{\mu}_{Yp\upsilon(q)} + \varepsilon_{Yp\upsilon(q)}\right)$$

where q identifies the criteria used for constructed confidence interval as follows

$q = 1$ if the normal approximation is accepted

$q = 2$ if the Parametric Boostrap is used

$q = 3$ if the Non-parametric Bootstrap is used

υ = separate product estimator, combined product estimator, separate imputation predictor, combined imputation predictor.

$\varepsilon_{Yp\upsilon(q)}$ is the semi-amplitude of the interval calculated using the corresponding method q for the estimator υ with $\alpha = 0.05$.

Experiment 1

We compared the different proposals developed in this paper using a data base provided from an experiment where the results for obtaining a recombinant protein production using fermentation in 786 samples. They are considered as a population and we identified the total protein in the liquid as the auxiliary variable X. The measured content of a protein is considered as Y. The non responses were considered for the samples which were re-evaluated due to technical problems. The results of interest for the estimation are given in the following table.

1,000 samples of size 80 were selected independently and the behavior of the estimations are in Table 5.18. The results establishes that to sub sample is better than to impute being the use of the Non Parametric Bootstrap the best alternative. The separate estimator is more reliable. The use of imputation using the separate criteria has a considerable better behavior. We compare the behavior of

$$\bar{y}_{ps} = \frac{n_1 \bar{y}_1 + n_2 \bar{y}'_{2p}}{n} = \frac{n_1 \bar{y}_1 + n_2 \bar{y}_2}{n} + \frac{n_2 (\bar{y}'_{2p} - \bar{y}_2)}{n},$$

$$\bar{y}_{pc} = \left(\frac{n_1 \bar{y}_1 + n_2 \bar{y}'_2}{n} \right) \frac{\bar{x}}{\mu_x}$$

Experiment 2

The other set of experiments consisted in the generation of 1,000 variables distributed according with the distributions normal, lognormal and exponential. Rueda et al. (2004) developed a similar experience for evaluating the behavior of some estimators of the mean when some observations were missing. We use the same parameters for generating variables distributed Normal and a lognormal variables with mean 4.9 and standard deviation 0.586. For the exponential the parameter was $\lambda = 4.9$. Once a variable was generated a Bernoulli experiment with parameter $W_2 = 0.372$ was performed. If the generated variable took the value one it was considered as a NR. The Monte Carlo procedure was used for evaluating the behavior of the estimators (Tables 5.19, 5.20).

5.4.3 Imputation in LRSS

In this section we analyze a simulation study for establishing the behavior of the imputation procedures proposed in Chap. 4. The experiments used six probability distribution functions. They are used usually in the evaluation of RSS strategies. 10,000 samples were generated and the accuracy of the estimates computed calculating the errors

Table 5.18 Evaluation of the proposals	Strata	W_i	Mean of the auxiliary variable	Variance of the auxiliary variable
	1	0.682	66.39	58.9
	2	0.372	131.83	16.2

Table 5.19 Percent of inclusion of the mean in 1,000 samples generated from a population of measurements of total and recombinant protein in fermentation experiments

Estimator	$q = 1$ Normal approximation	$q = 2, B = 20$ Parametric bootstrap	$q = 3, B = 20$ Non-parametric bootstrap
$\bar{y}_{ps}$	0.80	0.85	0.91
$\bar{y}_{pC}$	0.60	0.70	0.75
$\bar{y}_{Is}$	0.41	0.59	0.74
$\bar{y}_{IC}$	0.75	0.79	0.74

Table 5.20 Percent of inclusion of the mean in 1,000 samples generated from continuous variables

$N(4.9\ 0.586)$	$q = 1$ Normal approximation	$q = 2.\ B = 100$ Parametric boostrap	$q = 3.\ B = 100$ Non-parametric bootstrap
$\bar{y}_{ps}$	0.833	0.893	0.934
$\bar{y}_{pC}$	0.714	0.807	0.867
$\bar{y}_{Is}$	0.444	0.516	0.583
$\bar{y}_{IC}$	0.489	0.57	0.678
$logN(4.9\ 0.586)$	$q = 1$ Normal approximation	$q = 2.\ B = 20$ Parametric bootstrap	$q = 3.\ B = 20$ Non-parametric bootstrap
$\bar{y}_{ps}$	0.807	0.878	0.942
$\bar{y}_{pC}$	0.817	0.854	0.889
$\bar{y}_{Is}$	0.724	0.773	0.805
$\bar{y}_{IC}$	0.663	0.704	0.789
$Exp(4.9)$	$q = 1$ Normal approximation	$q = 2.\ B = 20$ Parametric bootstrap	$q = 3.\ B = 20$ Non-parametric bootstrap
$\bar{y}_{ps}$	0.740	0.788	0.923
$\bar{y}_{pC}$	0.627	0.711	0.887
$\bar{y}_{Is}$	0.533	0.655	0.714
$\bar{y}_{IC}$	0.454	0.559	0.674

$$A(e) = \frac{1}{10000} \sum_{s=1}^{10,000} |\hat{\mu} - \mu|_{s(e)} / \mu, e = \text{LRSS, LRSS}(M), R(\text{LRSS}), \text{LRSS}(R)$$

The overall sample size was $n = mr = 100$. A 10 % of non responses were generated at random.

Results of simulation, in terms of the accuracy, are summarized for $m = 4$ in Table 5.21. The differences between LRSS and the proposed estimator R(LRSS) are generally negligible, particularly for symmetric distributions. The use of the mean imputation, LRSS(M), seems to have a worse behavior, with respect to LRSS than LRSS(R) for R(LRSS).

A similar analysis is performed for $m = 5$ in Table 5.21. The differences between the full response estimators and the imputed are larger but the symmetry of the distributions seems to be important for establishing the existence of an adequate behavior of the imputation procedures (Tables 5.22, 5.23).

Table 5.21 Values of $A(e)$ for $m = 4$

Distribution	$m = 4$			
	LRSS	LRSS(M)	R(LRSS)	LRSS(R)
Uniform (0.1)	1.95	2.46	1.97	2.07
Normal (0.1)	1.34	3.46	1.37	2.19
Logistic (−1.1)	0.92	4.67	0.97	2.38
Exponential (1)	1.71	3.38	1.72	2.07
Exponential (2)	1.18	4.55	1.24	2.01
Gamma (1.2)	2.34	5.37	1.89	1.97
Ganma (2.1)	1.84	5.56	1.86	1.98
Weibull (1.3)	1.37	4.89	1.17	2.96
Weibull (3.1)	3.65	5.02	2.06	3.99

Table 5.22 Values of $A(e)$ for $m = 5$

Distribution	$m = 5$			
	LRSS	LRSS(M)	R(LRSS)	LRSS(R)
Uniform (0.1)	2.22	4.22	2.11	4.24
Normal (0.1)	2.34	3.97	2.28	4.01
Logistic (−1.1)	1.99	4.03	1.92	3.98
Exponential (1)	2.37	4.78	3.89	4.81
Exponential (2)	3.02	5.79	3.90	5.77
Gamma (1.2)	3.83	6.91	4.39	5.94
Gamma (2.1)	4.23	8.82	3.92	9.02
Weibull (1.3)	3.98	7.90	4.01	7.86
Weibull (3.1)	3.02	5.77	3.90	5.71

Table 5.23 Accuracy of the estimators for $m = 4, 5, 6, 7, 10, 11$

Method	Sample size					
	$m = 4$	$m = 5$	$m = 6$	$m = 7$	$m = 10$	$m = 11$
LRSS	1.180	2.213	2.995	3.158	3.228	4.004
LRSS(M)	2.887	2.889	3.895	3.970	3.905	4.180
R(LRSS)	1.230	2.551	3.001	3.322	3.452	3.974
LRSS(R)	2.008	2.676	3.152	3.405	3.615	3.912

The performance of the considered imputation methods is measured using the increment in the measurements of CO_2 in 250 monitoring stations. The ranking was made using the mean of the emission in the previous month in each of them. The mean $\mu = 1.056$ % and the variance $\sigma^2 = 89.33$. The skewness was of 1.794. Hence its distribution can not be considered symmetric. The simulation was made using different values of m for $r = 5$ and a 10 % of non responses were generated in each of the 10,000 simulated samples.

References

Al-Omari, A.I., Jaber,K., & Al-Omari, A. (2008). Modified ratio-type estimators of the mean using extreme ranked set sampling. *Journal of Mathematics and Statistics*, *4*, 150–155.

Al-Omari, A. I., Jemain, A. A., & Ibrahim, K. (2009). New ratio estimators of the mean using simple random sampling and ranked set sampling methods. *Revista Investigación Operacional*, *30*, 97–108.

Babu, C.J., & Singh, Y K. (1983). Non parametric inferences on means using bootstrap. Annals of Statistics, *11*, 999–1003.

Bhoj, D. S. (1997). Estimation of parameters of the extreme value distribution using ranked set sampling. *Communications in Statistics.-Theory and Methods, 26*, 653–662.

Bouza, C. N. (2001a). Model assisted ranked survey sampling. *Biometrical Journal, 43*, 249–259.

Bouza, C. N. (2001b). Ranked set sampling for estimating the differences of means. *Revista Investigación Operacional, 22*, 154–162.

Bouza, C. N. (2002A). Estimation of the mean in ranked set sampling with non responses. *Metrika, 56*, 171–179.

Bouza, C. N. (2002). Ranked set subsampling the non response strata for estimating the difference of mean. *Biometrical Journal, 44*, 903–915.

Bouza Herrera, C., & Schubert, L. (2003). The estimation of biodiversity and the characterization of the dynamics: an application to the study of a pest. Revista de Matematica E Estatistica, *21*, 85–98.

Castro, C. (2000). *Aportación estadística al conjoint analysis.* Tesis De Msc: Universidad De La Habana.

Chen, Z., Bai, Z., & Sinha, B.K. (2004). *Ranked set sampling: theory and applications. lecture notes in statistics*, (Vol. 176), Springer: New York.

Efron, B. (1979). Bootstrap methods : another look to the jacknife. *Annals Statistics, 7*, 1–26.

Laupracis, A., Sackett D.L., & Roberts R.S. (1988). An assesment of clinically useful measures of the consequences of treatment. *New England Journal of Medicine, 318*, 1728–1733.

Liu, L., Yujuan, T., Yingfu, L., & Guohua Z. (2006). Imputation for missing data and variance estimation when auxiliary information is incomplete. *Model Assisted Statistics and Applications, 1*, 83–94.

Little, R.J.A., & Rubin D.B. (1987). *Statistical analysis with missing data.* Wiley: New York.

Kadilar, C., & Cingi, H. (2008). Estimators for the population mean in the case of missing data. *Communication in Statistics-Theory and Methods, 37*, 2226–2236.

Muttlak, H. A. (1995). Median ranked set sampling. *Journal of Applied Statistical Science, 6*, 91–98.

Muttlak, H. A. (1998). Median ranked set sampling with size biased probability selection. *Biometrical Journal, 40*, 455–465.

Muttlak, H. A. (2001). Extreme ranked set sampling a comparison with regression and ranked set sampling. *Pakistan Journal of Statistics, 6*, 167–204.

Muttlak, H. A. (2003). Investigating the use of quartile ranked set samples for estimating the population mean. *Journal of Applied Mathematics and Computation, 146*, 437–445.

Parr, W. C. (1983). The bootstrap: some large sample theory and connections with robustness. *Statistics and Probability Letters, 3*, 97–100.

Rueda, M., & González, S. (2004). Missing data and auxiliary information in surveys. *Computational Statistics, 19*, 551–567.

Samawi, H., Abu-Dayyeh, W., & Ahmed, S. (1996a). Extreme ranked set sampling. *Biometrical Journal, 38*, 577–586.

Samawi, Hmandhamuttlak. (1996). Estimation of a ratio using ranked set sampling. *Biometrical Journal, 36*, 753–764.

Samawi, H.M., Ahmed, M.S., & Abu Dayyeh, W., (1996). Estimating the population mean using extreme ranked set sampling. *Biometrical Journal, 38*, 577–586.

Singh, S. & Deo, B. (20 03). Imputing with power transformation. *Statistical Papers, 44*, 555–579.

Viada González, C.E., Bouza Herrera, C.N., Torres Barbosa, F., & Torres Gemeil O., (2004). Estudio estadístico de ensayos clínicos de un medicamento para la psoriasis vulgar usando técnicas de imputación. *Revista Investigación Operacional, 25*, 243–255.

Index

C. N. Bouza-Herrera, *Handling Missing Data in Ranked Set Sampling*,   115
SpringerBriefs in Statistics, DOI: 10.1007/978-3-642-39899-5,
© The Author(s) 2013